Lifestyle Medicine From the Inside Out

Lifestyle Medicine From the Inside Out: Using Positive Psychology in Healthy Lifestyles for Positive Health summarizes the principles, science, and practice of how positive psychology can be integrated into lifestyle medicine for positive health in health care and self-care. This integration builds physical health and well-being, buffers against adversity, and promotes personal growth after traumatic experiences. By intertwining healthy habits and positive psychology-based activities, including personal strengths and what is meaningful to each person, individuals can truly thrive. Such an approach is what the authors refer to as practicing "lifestyle medicine from the inside out."

Co-authored by the lead developer of the original lifestyle medicine competencies, this book suggests positive health expansions for each competency, outlines specific questions that drive personal reflection for change and positive clinical interactions, and describes the step-by-step approach in case studies. Such innovative clinical practice that connects with what matters most to individuals is foundational to care.

In a rapidly changing and increasingly challenging world, health professionals in a wide variety of roles practicing in lifestyle medicine, primary care, and across medical specialties, patients, and all individuals can benefit from the insights and practical tips outlined in this book to achieve and maintain flourishing.

Liana S. Lianov, MD, MPH, is president and founder of the Global Positive Health Institute and Assistant Professor at the Centre for Positive Health, RCSI University of Medicine and Health Sciences, Ireland. She also serves as lead faculty for the American College of Lifestyle Medicine (ACLM) Physician and Health Professional Wellbeing course and Chair of the ACLM Happiness Science and Positive Health Committee and is ACLM past president.

Jolanta Burke is a Chartered Psychologist and Senior Lecturer (US: Associate Professor) at the Centre for Positive Health, RCSI University of Medicine and Health Sciences, Ireland.

Lifestyle Medicine From the Inside Out

Using Positive Psychology in Healthy Lifestyles for Positive Health

Liana S. Lianov and Jolanta Burke

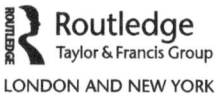

Routledge
Taylor & Francis Group

LONDON AND NEW YORK

Designed cover image: © Getty Images

First published 2025
by Routledge
4 Park Square, Milton Park, Abingdon, Oxon OX14 4RN

and by Routledge
605 Third Avenue, New York, NY 10158

Routledge is an imprint of the Taylor & Francis Group, an informa business

© 2025 Liana S. Lianov and Jolanta Burke

British Library Cataloguing-in-Publication Data
A catalog record for this book is available from the British Library

Library of Congress Cataloging-in-Publication Data
Names: Lianov, Liana S., author. | Burke, Jolanta, author.
Title: Lifestyle medicine from the inside out : using positive psychology in healthy lifestyles for positive health / Liana S. Lianov, and Jolanta Burke.
Description: Abingdon, Oxon ; New York, NY : Routledge, 2024. | Includes bibliographical references and index.
Identifiers: LCCN 2023057334 (print) | LCCN 2023057335 (ebook) | ISBN 9781032550749 (hardback) | ISBN 9781032550732 (paperback) | ISBN 9781003428909 (ebook)
Subjects: LCSH: Clinical health psychology. | Positive psychology. | Self-care, Health--Psychological aspects. | Lifestyles--Health aspects. | Health behavior.
Classification: LCC R726.7 .L543 2024 (print) | LCC R726.7 (ebook) | DDC 616.001/9--dc23/eng/20240319
LC record available at https://lccn.loc.gov/2023057334
LC ebook record available at https://lccn.loc.gov/2023057335

ISBN: 9781032550749 (hbk)
ISBN: 9781032550732 (pbk)
ISBN: 9781003428909 (ebk)

DOI: 10.4324/9781003428909

Typeset in Times New Roman
by KnowledgeWorks Global Ltd.

'*Lifestyle Medicine From the Inside Out: Using Positive Psychology in Healthy Lifestyles for Positive Health* provides a roadmap for a new paradigm in healthcare. Authored by thought leaders in positive health, it is a must read for health professionals looking for a better way to provide care.'

Darren Morton, *PhD, Director of the Lifestyle Medicine and Health Research Centre, Avondale University*

'Lifestyle medicine is the most exciting and important field in medicine today. *Lifestyle Medicine From the Inside Out* is an extraordinary book that shows us why and how to optimize it with positive psychology. Highly recommended.'

Dean Ornish, *MD, #1 New York Times bestselling author and Clinical Professor of Medicine, University of California, San Francisco*

'As I've matured in my practice of primary care using a lifestyle medicine foundation, it's become more and more clear to me that if I don't start with a deep and clear knowledge of each patient, approaching them from a wholistic perspective, and understanding their deep desires and sources of joy and happiness, then I can't be successful in influencing their lives. Liana Lianov has been instrumental in my journey towards providing the best of care and self-care to my patients. Now her wisdom, insights and vision are succinctly shared with us all in *Lifestyle Medicine From the Inside Out*. This book provides tools and resources, but perhaps more importantly it shares perspective, and that's something each of us needs in our lifestyle medicine journey. Yes, we are reversing disease, but more importantly, we're healing whole people.'

Wayne S. Dysinger, *MD, MPH, Physician and Founder, Lifestyle Medical*

'*Lifestyle Medicine From the Inside Out* explores the six pillars of lifestyle medicine through the lens of positive psychology concepts. This book also outlines the core competencies of lifestyle medicine, providing positive health expansions for each competency. It is a wonderful addition to the books on lifestyle medicine and positive health that can help transform health and healthcare.'

Beth Frates, *MD, President of the American College of Lifestyle Medicine; Assistant Professor, Part-Time, Harvard Medical School*

'A very timely publication and call to action which considers the complexity of the challenges faced by humanity and the role that lifestyle medicine can play in navigating our course.'

Professor Karen Morgan, *President and CEO, RCSI and UCD Malaysia Campus*

'Lianov and Burke have found the warm, beating heart of Lifestyle Medicine. They masterfully guide the reader toward thriving, positive health for themselves and their patients.'

Edward M Phillips, *MD, Associate Professor, Physical Medicine and Rehabilitation, Harvard Medical School. Author of* Food, We Need to Talk: The science-based, humor-laced last word on eating, diet and making peace with your body *(2023)*

Contents

1 The Evolution of Positive Psychology, Lifestyle Medicine, and Positive Health

Chapter Overview

This chapter introduces the practice of lifestyle medicine and its pillars – healthy eating, physical activity, sleep, avoidance of risky substance use, stress management, and social connection – and potential role of positive psychology interventions. We also introduce positive psychology, its early history, evolution of theories, and current state of the field and how it is being integrated with lifestyle medicine for positive health.

The Emergence of Positive Psychology to Advance Health and Wellbeing

Health sciences are primarily concerned with treatment and prevention. The same approach has been prevalent in other fields, such as psychology, neuroscience, leadership, or education. By the late 1990s, barely 1.5% of research papers delved into what is right with people, their positive subjective experiences, such as wellbeing, and how individuals could not only prevent illness but thrive (Rusk & Waters, 2013). This imbalance of research had consequences for how we understood human beings. For example, we learned about a healthy brain by studying what people with dementia could not do. As such, we could only guess what the healthy brain looked like and assumed that a healthy brain was an optimally performing brain, which is a fallacy. Just because people are not sick does not mean they are happy or healthy, and it certainly does not mean they are thriving. A more balanced perspective was required, which is what positive psychology advocated.

Positive psychology emerged in 1988 when Prof Martin Seligman became the president of the American Psychological Association (Seligman, 1988). Like all presidents before him, he stood on the podium before his peers and proclaimed what, in his opinion, were the limitations of the psychology field

DOI: 10.4324/9781003428909-1

and what he wanted to address during his presidency. He focused on the deficit approach to human beings that permeated psychological research. He talked about psychology becoming a healing profession that helped a select few rather than the science that made all people's lives better. He talked about the research and practice of becoming primarily focused on what is wrong with people, not what is right, and the need to research human strengths that complement the Diagnostic and Statistical Manual of Mental Disorders (DSM). That day, modern positive psychology was launched and has since grown exponentially.

Positive psychology was not a new field of science. The term positive psychology was first introduced by a humanistic psychologist Abraham Maslow (1954). The topics positive psychology covers reach as far back as the publications at the end of the 19th century by the father of psychology, William James. Over the last century, many researchers have studied topics under positive psychology. In the 1960s and 1970s, some foundations for positive psychology emerged, such as research about self-efficacy, happiness, love, and positive emotions, to mention a few. However, it was scarce. For example, before the launch of positive psychology, the ratio of articles about depression and happiness was 17:1 (Achor, 2010). Similarly, neuropsychological research constituted barely 7% of articles about the positive aspects of the brain, with the vast majority focusing on deficits (Randolph, 2013). According to Carl Rogers's theory, more research was required to understand the whole person.

In the first decade of positive psychology, the main focus of research was to highlight the positive aspects of human beings, their experience, and outcomes (Seligman & Csikszentmihalyi, 2000). Specifically, it focused on positive subjective experiences like happiness, contentment, and compassion. Researchers were also exploring positive aspects of individuals, such as character strengths. Finally, it included research on how positive organizations, such as hospitals, facilitated individuals' and teams' optimal states. Thus, to help positive psychology establish the field, it initially focused on differentiating itself by focusing on the positives.

However, soon it was criticized for encouraging "the tyranny of positive thinking" (Held, 2002) and lack of scientific rigor. For example, Sonya Lyubomirsky's "happiness pie," which was once used extensively to convince people to practice positive psychology interventions, was discredited by genetic researchers. According to the model, 40% of wellbeing depends on intentional activity, 10% on circumstances, and a further 50% on genetics (Lyubomirsky et al., 2005). However, given the emergence of epigenetics that explores the impact of the environment on gene expression, the pie was perceived as too simplistic, and its main components were questioned (Brown & Rohrer, 2020). The researchers acknowledged that the impact of interventions had been overestimated, and their updated thinking offered a more balanced perspective (Sheldon & Lyubomirsky, 2021).

Similarly, Barbara Fredrickson's research on positive emotions evolved into quantifying a ratio of 5:1 of positive and negative emotional experiences leading to psychological flourishing (Fredrickson & Losada, 2005). However, the algorithm used for assessing the ratio was challenged by other researchers (Brown et al., 2013), leading to Fredrickson withdrawing the ratio findings and acknowledging the remaining aspects of her theory that were based on rigorous science (Fredrickson, 2013).

The challenges experienced by researchers approximately a decade after the launch of positive psychology became a building block of future rigorous research in the field. More careful study designs that ensured the accuracy of the findings have emerged. European and Canadian researchers called for the second wave of positive psychology that explores not only the positive aspects of human traits and experiences but also how negativity can become a building block for positive outcomes (Lomas & Ivtzan, 2016; Wang, 2015). This research included examining trauma as a springboard for posttraumatic growth or exploring the adaptive role of sadness and other negative emotions. The second wave of positive psychology embraced all human experiences, including suffering and their pathways for positive outcomes.

Since then, a third wave of positive psychology has emerged (Lomas et al., 2021). It acknowledges the complexities of human beings beyond the dichotomous positive versus negative perspectives. It examines positive psychology in the context of multidisciplinary research, such as connecting health and positive psychology. It also explores alternative methodologies for research that go beyond the post-positivist perspective of hard-core quantitative research favoring randomized control trials. This way, a more balanced approach is developed

Even more importantly, the landscape of positive psychology research is rapidly changing. In the first wave of positive psychology, US-led research was predominant. However, nowadays, most of the research published in positive psychology comes from outside the United States (Kim et al., 2018). Its influence extends to Europe, Asia, the Americas, Oceania, and Africa. Even though research continues to be predominantly WEIRD, i.e., conducted with white, educated individuals from industrialized, prosperous, and democratic countries (Hendriks et al., 2019), systematically, more research is conducted with diverse populations. Thus, positive psychology is no longer an extension of the American dream, but a solid field of research that explores the good life worldwide. This is no surprise, as positive psychology aligns with ancient wisdom that arose in cultures and nations outside of the United States, for example, as part of Eastern philosophy and related practices.

At the same time, positive psychology continues to explore ways in which the field can grow and improve based on the latest criticisms that continue to emerge (van Zyl et al., 2023). Bringing positive psychological knowledge into lifestyle medicine can enrich both fields. What is essential is to keep a critical perspective when merging these two types of science, which is what this book aims to do.

The Emergence of Lifestyle Medicine

In the early 2000s the term "lifestyle medicine" was used by a small group of practitioners applying healthy lifestyles as a primary treatment. The American College of Lifestyle Medicine (ACLM) was formed in 2004 to advance the emerging field. However, most healthcare practitioners were unaware of the term or defined it in different ways. The lack of a standard definition represented a barrier to effective communication about relevant research and clinical application. Therefore, in 2009, leaders of the ACLM and the American College of Preventive Medicine (ACPM) convened a panel of representatives from an array of medical specialty societies to define lifestyle medicine and identify the knowledge and skills that physicians need to offer high-quality clinical services. The consensus panel led by Mark Johnson and Liana Lianov developed a definition for lifestyle medicine and 15 core competencies for primary care physicians later expanded to other health professionals (Lianov & Johnson, 2010).

The panel defined lifestyle medicine as "The evidence-based practice of helping individuals and families adopt and sustain healthy behaviors that affect health and quality of life." This definition reflects the panelists' emphasis on supporting patients with behavior change as the root of the practice to optimize health outcomes. The fundamentals of lifestyle medicine emphasize science-based healthy lifestyle interventions, team-based care, behavioral science, and patient and family/caregiver support enhanced with community resources.

The core competencies developed through the alignment of the panel of representatives from diverse physicians and health organizations marked the birth of the new field of lifestyle medicine. Provider self-care was highlighted as an essential competency area to prevent clinician burnout or distress and enhance providers' lifestyle counseling.

The statement of the consensus panel was published in the *Journal of the American Medical Association* on July 14, 2010, and nudged the general medical community to adopt these competencies. In 2013, an ACLM National Standards Task Force added the domains stress management and "interpersonal-community-group relationships" to modalities identified by the panel of nutrition, physical activity, and sleep identified by the original panel. Hence, key pillars of practice have evolved and now included a predominant-plant based eating pattern, physical activity, restorative sleep, tobacco cessation and avoidance of risky substance use, stress management, and social connection, which we address in this book.

Organizations and partners in addition to the ACLM, such as the Institute of Lifestyle Medicine, have contributed to training health professionals in the US, and the ever-expanding number of lifestyle medicine organizations globally provide training and support to practitioners. Moreover, the American Board of Lifestyle Medicine founded in 2017 and later the International Board of Lifestyle Medicine were formed to offer a standardized examination and certification in the field. These organizations are bringing positive psychology into the field.

Linking Lifestyle Medicine with Positive Psychology for Positive Health

Although at first sight there is minimal similarity between the two fields, they are interdependent. Lifestyle medicine focuses on treating chronic diseases; positive psychology focuses on how to help people experience optimal human functioning. Yet, both fields are interconnected in a range of ways.

Complementary Relationship

One way to perceive the relationship between both fields is by seeing it as complementary (Figure 1.1).

Both fields have contributed to creating knowledge and guidance on the best practices associated with being healthy. Lifestyle medicine provides in-depth insights into treating and reversing disease, as well as keeping bodies healthy by eating well, engaging in physical activity, sleeping well, and managing stress and substances. It also taps into the social aspect of human needs by exploring relationships. On the other hand, positive psychology explores states and conditions of a good life that contribute to optimal human functioning. Both approaches are needed for individuals to live a good life. If they do not get a good night's sleep, their mood will dampen. To improve their mood, they can either go to bed earlier (if sleep hygiene is the issue) or practice positive psychology interventions (if the mental state is the issue for not getting a good night's sleep). Thus, using the knowledge from both fields can help individuals maximize their health and wellbeing outcomes.

Another way both fields complement each other relates to the body and mind perspectives. Lifestyle medicine may be seen as concerned mainly with the body. Positive psychology is often perceived as a head-up approach (Hefferon, 2013) because it focuses on the psyche and ways; we can change the mind to experience optimal human functioning. Thus, the mutual approach of acknowledging a person as comprising both and considering the impact that it may have on wellbeing is crucial.

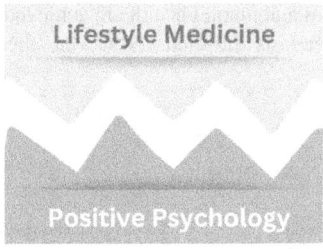

Figure 1.1 A graphical representation of the complementary relationship between lifestyle medicine and positive psychology.

Interdependence of the Fields

The impact of each field on both body and mind is increasingly evident. Moreover, the positive psychology has an essential role in a successful medical practice that relies on behavior change. Health coaches have incorporated positive psychology as a key technique along with motivational interviewing and cognitive behavior change. Other health team members are beginning to apply positive psychology constructs into care, such as focusing on what is meaningful to the patient. Using both lifestyle change and positive psychology can address both physical and mental health needs.

Case Study

Stephen had prostate cancer surgical treatment several months ago. After his diagnosis, he started to experience anxiety and depression, which stayed with him despite taking a selective serotonin reuptake inhibitor medication. He wants to get his overall health back on track. He works with his health practitioner to develop a health action plan that will support both his physical health condition and improve his mental and emotional wellbeing. They create a program intertwining lifestyle medicine and positive psychology interventions, including increased walking intensity, increased fruit and vegetable consumption, and a gratitude journal. The health coach uses motivational interviewing and positive psychology techniques to help Stephan with achieving the action plan.

Expansive Relationship

Both fields may also be perceived as having an expansive relationship with each other (Figure 1.2).

The focus of lifestyle medicine is treatment, as well as prevention, of disease. When physical and mental health are achieved, the role of the practitioner may be viewed as fulfilled. However, the positive psychology

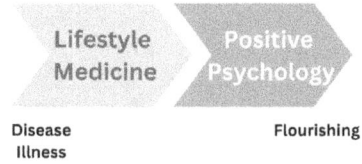

Disease   Flourishing
Illness

Figure 1.2 A graphical representation of the expansive relationship between lifestyle medicine and positive psychology.

perspective considers the need to go beyond illness focus to a wellbeing focus. It is not enough to get rid of disease; we need to aim to go beyond the latter. While a plant-based eating pattern and regular physical activity can prevent and treat obesity, to truly flourish, we need to incorporate the healthy lifestyle pillars with positive psychology approaches. This will ensure that our body and mind are healthy and that we are thriving by engaging in a range of additional behaviors that will support the whole person going forward.

Case Study

Trudy lived a good life. She ate mostly plant-based whole foods, went for a 30-minute run most mornings, kept her stress in check with mindfulness practices, and slept well. She did not overuse substances and had several friends she could rely on. Despite all this, her life felt empty. She could not understand it, as she was healthy and did well in all the six pillars of lifestyle medicine. To move it up a level, she needed a change. She decided she would start introducing positive activities (such as focusing on what she finds meaningful) for 10 minutes each day. They will help her determine what she values and do more of what makes her happy. Within a month, she found bounce in her step, and her life became more enjoyable.

Maximizing Relationship

Maximizing relationship relates to getting the best out of people so that they can use positive psychology to fully engage in lifestyle medicine and they can use lifestyle medicine to maximize their health and wellbeing (Figure 1.3).

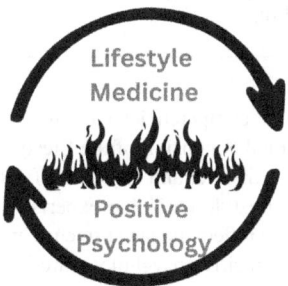

Figure 1.3 A graphical representation of the maximizing relationship between lifestyle medicine and positive psychology.

The fields can maximize each other's outcomes. For example, techniques drawn from positive psychology could make engaging in physical activity more effective. Equally, physical activity engagement could support individuals in managing their mood. Therefore, both fields can complement each other, and their results can be maximized when applied together.

Case Study

Mandy consumed too much alcohol every day. She was aware of it but could not stop herself from drinking. Every night after work, she opened a bottle, sat in front of the TV, and tried to forget about her busy day. Thoughts ran fast through her mind: snippets of conversations with colleagues, a flashback to the to-do list for the next day, or the feeling overwhelmed she felt at work.

She decided to reduce her drinking by not consuming alcohol during the weekday, only reaching out for it over the weekend. However, as soon as she began the process, another problem emerged. Without her glass of wine, she could not relax in the evening. If she managed to forget about work by distracting herself with a TV program or a computer game, as soon as her head hit the pillow, so had the flashbacks that kept her awake for hours. She needed to do something extra to maximize her effectiveness.

She opted for positive psychology interventions. During her morning shower, she thought of three enjoyable things she would do that day. After work, before heading home, she wrote down her deepest thoughts and feelings about the day, focusing on what went well for her and what she would address the next day. She left her diary behind, so by the time she got home, she did not need to suppress any thoughts associated with work; she just focused her attention on the here and now. This is how her use of positive psychology interventions has aided her goal to reduce alcohol.

The lifestyle medicine competencies were updated in 2022 (Lianov et al., 2022) with a more detailed expansion of the lifestyle modalities and included positive psychology as a distinct and key area of successful practice. A committee of international lifestyle medicine experts will continue to update the competencies regularly to reflect the latest science and the advancing standards of the field. Elements of positive psychology are included at its core. Of note, although the field of lifestyle medicine is not fully maximizing positive psychology, some early adopters are integrating it into medicine, and some view

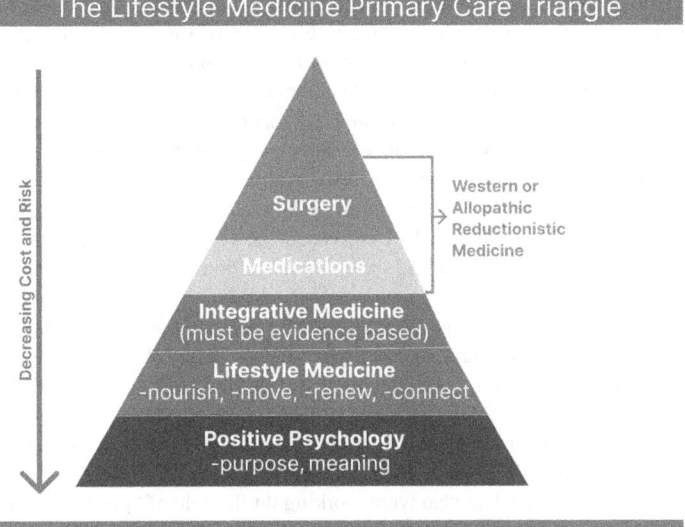

Figure 1.4 Lifestyle medicine primary care pyramid containing positive psychology at the base (shown with permission from Wayne Dysinger MD).

it as the foundation to successful care. Figure 1.4 is an example developed by Wayne Dysinger, who received the Trailblazer Award from the ACLM.

The Evolution of Positive Health by Integrating Lifestyle Medicine, Positive Psychology, and the Person-Centered Whole Health Approach

Lifestyle medicine is evolving in its focus on person-centered whole health care, which emphasizes motivation and empowering the individual in their personalized care with the support of trusted relationships with the health team to facilitate patient-driven action that treat disease and promote wellbeing.

Emotional and mental wellbeing is the heart of a person's capacity to achieve and sustain healthy lifestyles. Emotional distress and mood disorders are seen as frequent comorbidities to common chronic illnesses, such as diabetes and cardiovascular diseases, and decrease successful health behavior changes. The role and effectiveness of interventions, such as mindfulness-based stress reduction, have increasingly been recognized. Skills at applying screening tools for stress, depression, and anxiety, assisting patients with self-management, and implementing positive psychology approaches have garnered increasing attention. Effective patient relationships, referred to as the therapeutic alliance, are viewed as foundational to the person-centered approach and were added to the 2022 competencies. Also, wellbeing and positive psychology have been identified as essential. Studies support that positive psychology interventions have a statistically significant small to moderate effect on psychological and subjective wellbeing quality of life, strengths, depression, anxiety, and stress (Carr, et al., 2023) – which impact healthy lifestyle behaviors. The ACLM convened the Happiness Science in Health Care Summit in 2018, leading to recommendations for further research and application.

Other groups have also recognized the role of positive psychology in health and in health care, for example with the establishment of the Center for Positive Psychology and Health at the RCSI University of Medical and Health Sciences in 2019. This work on positive psychology and health is being shaped to harness the broader biopsychosocial model with the construct of "positive health," which does not yet have a standard definition. Health and psychology leaders also were working on the role of "positive health" in medical care. One of these groups was the Institute of Positive Health, led by Machteld Huber, which convened a summit on positive health in 2009 and has been conducting positive health trainings globally. The Global Positive Health Institute (GPHI) was founded in 2020, emphasizing the link between lifestyle medicine, positive psychology, and the broader biopsychosocial model as foundational to health care for best outcomes. The GPHI offers positive health education and practice tools to health professionals. The Center for Positive Health Sciences at the Royal College of Surgeons Ireland (RCSI) University of Medical and Health Sciences is conducting innovative research and providing leading-edge education to health professional trainees. Although the use of the term 'positive health' by such groups varies somewhat, major underlying principles are aligned.

Positive health, as we use it here, is both a journey toward wellbeing via this clinical and self-care approach and a destination of becoming one's best self regardless of underlying mental and physical conditions. In this model that contains two-continua (Figure 1.5), progress can be made on the positive health continuum independently of getting rid of disease, yet such progress can influence behavior change and even lead to direct physical benefits along the illness continuum. Integrating lifestyle and positive psychology approaches helps patients move along the positive health continuum, while also influencing progress on the illness continuum, with improved treatment adherence and direct physiologic benefits. The next several chapters focus on how each healthy lifestyle can be combined with positive psychology for such positive health results.

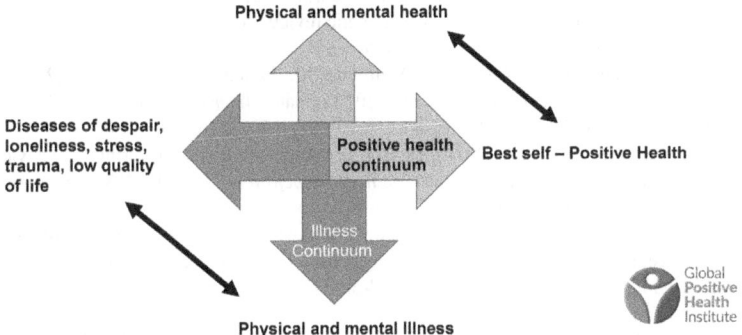

Figure 1.5 A graphic representation of medical practice that combines both an illness and a positive health continuum (copyrighted and shown with permission from the Global Positive Health Institute).

References

Achor, S. (2010). *The happiness advantage: The seven principles of positive psychology that fuel success and performance at work.* Crown Business/Random House. https://doi.org/10.1007/s10943-020-01146-w

Brown, N. J. L., & Rohrer, J. M. (2020). Easy as (happiness) pie? A critical evaluation of a popular model of the determinants of well-being. *Journal of Happiness Studies: An Interdisciplinary Forum on Subjective Well-Being, 21*(4), 1285–1301. https://doi.org/10.1007/s10902-019-00128-4.

Brown, N. J. L., Sokal, A. D., & Friedman, H. L. (2013). The complex dynamics of wishful thinking: The critical positivity ratio. *American Psychologist, 68*(9), 801–813. https://doi.org/10.1037/a0032850.

Carr, A., Finneran, L., Boyd., C., Shirey, C., Canning, C., Stafford, O., Lyons, J., Cullen, K., Prendergast, C., Corbett, C., Drumm, C, & Burke, T. The evidence-based for positive psychology interventions: a mega-analysis of meta-analyses. *The Journal of Positive Psychology.* 19(2), 191–205. https://doi.org/10.1080/17439760.2023.2168564

Fredrickson, B. L., & Losada, M. F. (2005). Positive affect and the complex dynamics of human flourishing. *American Psychologist, 60*(7), 678–686. https://doi.org/10.1037/0003-066X.60.7.678.

Fredrickson, B. L. (2013). Positive emotions broaden and build. In P. Devine & A. Plant (Eds.). *Advances in Experimental Social Psychology, 47,* 1–53, Burlington: Academic Press. https://doi.org/10.1016/B978-0-12-407236-7.00001-2

Hefferon, K. (2013). *Positive body: Somatopsychic wellbeing.* Open University Press.

Held, B. S. (2002). The negative side of positive psychology. *Journal of Humanistic Psychology,* 44(1). https://doi.org/10.1177/0022167803259645

Hendriks, T., Warren, M. A., Schotanus-Dijkstra, M., Hassankhan, A., Graafsma, T., Bohlmeijer, E., & de Jong, J. (2019). How WEIRD are positive psychology interventions? A bibliometric analysis of randomized controlled trials on the science of well-being. *The Journal of Positive Psychology, 14*(4), 489–501. https://doi.org/10.1080/17439760.2018.1484941.

Kim, H., Doiron, K., Warren, M., & Donaldson, S. (2018). The international landscape of positive psychology research: A systematic review. *International Journal of Wellbeing, 8*(1). https://doi.org/10.5502/ijw.v8i1.651

Lianov, L., Adamson, K., Kelly, J. H., Matthews, M., Palma, M., & Rea, B. L. (2022). Lifestyle medicine core competencies: 2022 update. *American Journal of Lifestyle Medicine, 16*(6), 734–739. https://doi.org/10.1177/15598276221121580.

Lianov, L., & Johnson, M. (2010). Physician competencies for prescribing lifestyle medicine. *Journal of the American Medical Association*, 304, 202–203. https://doi.org/10.1001/jama.2010.903

Lomas, T., & Ivtzan, I. (2016). Second wave positive psychology: Exploring the positive–negative dialectics of wellbeing. *Journal of Happiness Studies: An Interdisciplinary Forum on Subjective Well-Being, 17*(4), 1753–1768. https://doi.org/10.1007/s10902-015-9668-y.

Lomas, T., Waters, L., Williams, P., Oades, L. G., & Kern, M. L. (2021). Third wave positive psychology: Broadening towards complexity. *The Journal of Positive Psychology, 16*(5), 660–674. https://doi.org/10.1080/17439760.2020.1805501.

Lyubomirsky, S., Sheldon, K. M., & Schkade, D. (2005). Pursuing happiness: The architecture of sustainable change. *Review of General Psychology, 9*(2), 111–131. https://doi.org/10.1037/1089-2680.9.2.111.

Maslow, A. H. (1954). *Motivation and personality*. Harper.

Randolph, J. J. (2013). What is positive neuropsychology? In J. J. Randolph (Ed.), *Positive neuropsychology: Evidence-based perspectives in promoting cognitive health* (pp. 1–11). Springer Science and Business Media. https://doi.org/10.1007/978-1-4614-6605-5_1

Rusk, R. D., & Waters, L. E. (2013). Tracing the size, reach, impact, and breadth of positive psychology. *The Journal of Positive Psychology, 8*(3), 207–221. https://doi.org/10.1080/17439760.2013.777766.

Seligman, M. E., & Csikszentmihalyi, P. (2000). Positive psychology: An introduction. *American Psychologist, 55*(1), 5–14. https://doi.org/10.1037/0003-066X.55.1.5.

Seligman, M. E. P. (1998). The president's address. *American Psychologist, 54*, 559–562.

Sheldon, K. M., & Lyubomirsky, S. (2021). Revisiting the sustainable happiness model and pie chart: Can happiness be successfully pursued? *The Journal of Positive Psychology, 16*(2), 145–154. https://doi.org/10.1080/17439760.2019.1689421.

van Zyl, L. E., Gaffaney, J., van der Vaart, L., Dik, B. J., & Donaldson, S. I. (2023). The critiques and criticisms of positive psychology: A systematic review. *The Journal of Positive Psychology*. Advance Online Publication. https://doi.org/10.1080/17439760.2023.2178956.

Wang, Y., Wang, X., Yang, J., Zeng, P., & Lei, L. (2020). Body talk on social networking sites, body surveillance, and body shame among young adults: The roles of self-compassion and gender. *Sex Roles: A Journal of Research, 82*, 731–742. https://doi.org/10.1007/s11199-019-01084-2.

2 Wellbeing Theories and the Application of Positive Psychology

Chapter Overview

This chapter introduces positive psychology interventions and their application for wellbeing and positive health, which can be achieved when integrated with healthy lifestyles. Major wellbeing models, including the PERMA model, the flourishing in Europe model, and the mental health continuum model, summarized here can be used to develop frameworks of clinical and self-care with wellbeing interventions. These interventions leverage main concepts in positive psychology, such as character strengths, hope and optimism, positive emotions, and meaning in life.

Introduction

In this text, we focus on the science and practice of applying positive psychology with each of the lifestyle medicine pillars. We introduce the positive health approach that sees positive psychology as foundational to medical care. For positive health outcomes, we leverage the reinforcing link between these fields and integrate these approaches for health behavior change and direct physiologic benefits from physical and positive psychology-based activities. The first part reviews the science, the second provides practical implementation guidance, and the third summarizes the models of care that can best harness positive health, highlights the science showing impact of positive psychology on major chronic diseases, and makes recommendations for future research and health practice and health system change.

Positive Psychology Interventions (PPIs) in Action

If you ask anyone what they truly value, they usually point to health and wellbeing. This is why the global personal development market has exceeded

DOI: 10.4324/9781003428909-2

€40 billion a year, and it is anticipated to grow an additional 5% year-on-year between 2023 and 2030 (Grand View Research, 2023). Every day, millions of social media posts, self-help publications, and smartphone apps encourage people to engage with the latest health and wellbeing tools, many of which are informed by positive psychology research.

The positive psychology field prides itself on its research translation and application. The most prevalent application of positive psychology relates to PPIs, which are evidence-based activities that not only reduce adverse outcomes, such as negative affect, depression, or anxiety, but also show evidence of improving positive outcomes, such as increasing positive affect, engagement, or self-acceptance (Parks & Biswas Diener, 2013). They include activities such as "counting your blessings," "acts of kindness," "savoring," or "humor-inducing."

Even though PPIs are widely popular and often applied in a range of fields, such as psychotherapy, education, the workplace, and increasingly in healthcare, the complexity of their design contributes to their increased effectiveness (Parks & Biswas Diener, 2013). That complexity relates to exploring what their desired positive outcome may be. For example, in some cases, they are designed to improve happiness, meaning in life, and success at reaching goals. In other cases, when applied in healthcare, their positive outcome may be medication adherence, sustaining healthy behavior, or improving mental health, which supports individuals' physical health.

Apart from the desired positive outcome, each PPI targets a specific system, the domain within which a change occurs. The systems range from changing affect to more positive (e.g. practicing self-compassion), refocusing individuals' attention (e.g. reflecting on three good things after a surgery), or activating memory to instigate change (e.g. reminiscing of the good old times). Within healthcare, that targeting could also relate to physiological and health behavior systems, such as heart rate variability (e.g. encouraging individuals to connect with nature) and posture (e.g. practicing self-regulation). Thus, each PPI may be designed or tested to target one or many systems.

The target system aims to instigate change; as such, each intervention is designed to target a specific change that may benefit individuals and contribute to the desired outcome. For example, that target change may be self-esteem (e.g. to help individuals believe they can take action to lose weight), self-determination (e.g. to help individuals find the motivation to keep going during cancer treatment), social responsivity (e.g. to help individuals connect with their community), or hope (e.g. to create the will and the way for chronic disease management).

Once the desired outcomes, target system, and change are established, each intervention comprises at least one active ingredient that causes the change that could be questioned (e.g. asking participants what the benefit of their illness is), mindfulness (e.g. savoring the moment), or disputation (e.g. challenging their pessimistic thoughts). Each activity comprises a set of actions that could influence the outcome. As such, researchers often "play" around to see which action is more effective in inducing the targeted change. For example, that action could be writing (e.g. write a letter of forgiveness to someone who did you wrong), thinking about something (e.g. think of unique ways in which you could use your strengths next week), or taking action (e.g. perform three small acts of kindness today).

Therefore, the elements that PPIs comprise are essential to PPI effectiveness. They can either reduce or improve the targeted outcomes. They can also ease the application of PPIs in healthcare. For example, due to some physical or psychological limitations, patients may be unable to complete writing activities. However, they could instead think of something, move in a certain way, or say something. It is up to the patient and healthcare professional to decide. Furthermore, PPI practice has cultural differences (Layous et al., 2013). Flexibility should be practiced in applying the interventions and matching them to individuals (Li et al., 2021). It is often done on a trial-and-error basis; thus, working closely with patients is essential.

Researchers from the RCSI University of Medicine and Health Sciences have recently reviewed the literature and compiled over 100 evidence-based tools that combined PPIs with the six pillars of lifestyle medicine (Burke et al., 2023a). The inclusion criteria for the interventions included:

1 Presence of positive outcomes, e.g. aspects of health and wellbeing
2 Evidence of reducing illness (mental and physical)
3 Evidence of both psychological and physiological effects on wellbeing

All interventions that comprised the three categories were included. Burke et al. (2023b) have further developed this by coining the term positive health interventions (PHI), defined as "tools that aim to build psychological, emotional, intellectual, physiological and social resources that not only demonstrate the evidence of improving health and wellbeing, but also a reduction in the burden of disease." These tools included positive psychological activities that showed evidence of impacting sleep (e.g. listening to music before bed), physical activity (e.g. using character strengths to engage in exercise), or nutrition (e.g. eating more than seven fruit and vegetables a day associated with the highest levels of wellbeing) and all other pillars of lifestyle medicine.

In addition to using PPIs to directly impact positive outcomes, positive psychology wellbeing models can be used to structure a conversation, a clinical approach, or self-care for healthcare professionals. Wellbeing models guide what positive psychological outcomes can support individuals to improve wellbeing, prevent mental health issues, and support them in maximizing their engagement in lifestyle medicine pillars. Our latest research showed that in 1,112 participants, those who reported the highest levels of wellbeing were nine times more likely to use more than three pillars of lifestyle medicine than those who reported poor mental health (Burke & Dunne, 2022).

Thus, wellbeing models and lifestyle medicine are inextricably linked and can leveraged for positive health.

Wellbeing Models

Wellbeing is one of the most confusing terms, in that it can be understood as the absence of disease, illness, or disorder (e.g. anxiety, depression, Crohn's) and the presence of resources that support the good life (e.g. autonomy, personal growth, or optimism). The positive psychology perspective focuses on exploring the conditions and resources that help individuals live good lives, prevent them from experiencing some diseases, or ease their disease symptoms (Burke & Dunne, 2022). As such, it explores very different topics that most clinical or health psychologists would explore. Furthermore, positive psychology examines specific topics and offers unique suggestions for improving people's health and wellbeing.

Over the years, two main models of wellbeing emerged, the hedonic and eudaimonic wellbeing. They derived from distinct philosophical perspectives. Hedonism places an important value on experiencing pleasure and avoiding pain (Fletcher, 2016). Thus, they engage in a push-and-pull action, whereby individuals constantly aim to seek out more pleasure to reduce pain. Eudaimonia is about the pursuit of a virtuous life that is irrespective of pleasure. Psychological research has advanced the understanding of hedonic and eudaimonic wellbeing when it explored them empirically and created psychological tests for them.

Hedonic wellbeing is nowadays synonymous with happiness and is sometimes referred to as emotional or subjective wellbeing (SWB), as the theory emerged following interviews with the happiest people who shared their SWB experiences. SWB comprises three elements: (1) higher levels of positive emotions, (2) lower levels of negative emotions, and (3) higher levels of life satisfaction (Diener et al., 2017). In practice, it meant that happy people were regularly engaged in activities that brought them such positive emotions as joy, excitement, connection, or serenity. They also knew how to manage their negative emotions, e.g. sadness and anxiousness, effectively so that they did not overwhelm them. Finally, the life satisfaction component was associated with a positive evaluation of their lives. When asked to assess life satisfaction, individuals usually think of where they hoped to be now and then assess if they are already there. If what they hoped has come true, they are satisfied with their lives; if it has not yet, their satisfaction is reduced. However, the challenge with life satisfaction is that it often depends on our mood (Kahneman & Riis, 2005), and, hence, more accurate assessments are needed.

Eudaimonic wellbeing has been explored in psychology across various models and concepts. However, the most popular is the psychological wellbeing model, inspired by a century of research conducted by Allport, Maslow, Jung, Frankl, and many other psychologists exploring the good life.

It comprises six components of wellbeing: positive relations, meaning and purpose, autonomy, environmental mastery (knowing we can make changes in our lives), personal growth, and self-acceptance (Roepke et al., 2014). The hedonic and eudaimonic models competed with each other for a couple of decades until the launch of the new science of positive psychology that aimed to contribute to this research and practice.

With the emergence of positive psychology, a new model of authentic happiness was developed (Seligman & Csikszentmihalyi, 2000). It combined the latest, at the time, research on the importance of positive emotions with eudaimonic elements of engagement, meaning, and purpose. However, the model was re-evaluated a decade later and turned into the currently salient wellbeing model, commonly known as PERMA (Seligman, 2002). PERMA stands for Positive emotions, Engagement, Relationships, Meaning, and Accomplishment. Nowadays, a range of PERMA versions exists, such as adding H for Health to the five essential components (Figure 2.1).

The PERMA model was inspired by researchers from the University of Cambridge, who explored the highest levels of wellbeing (flourishing) with over 60,000 European citizens (Huppert & So, 2013). Their conceptualization of wellbeing comprised five core elements (positive emotions, engagement,

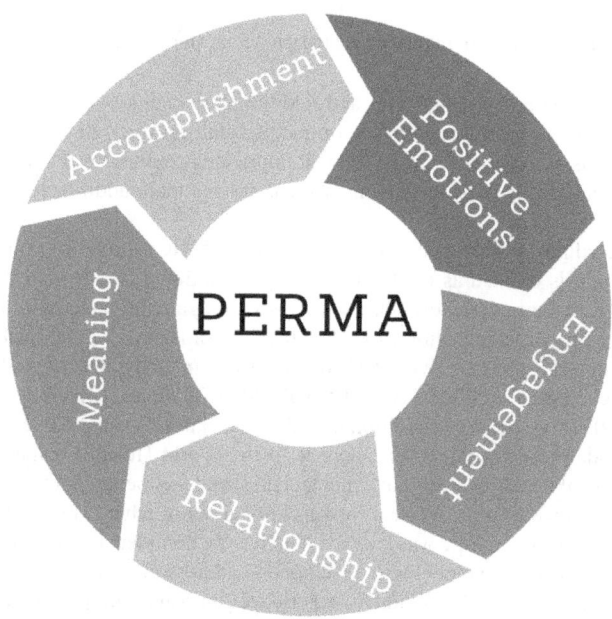

Figure 2.1 PERMA model (adapted from Seligman, 2011).

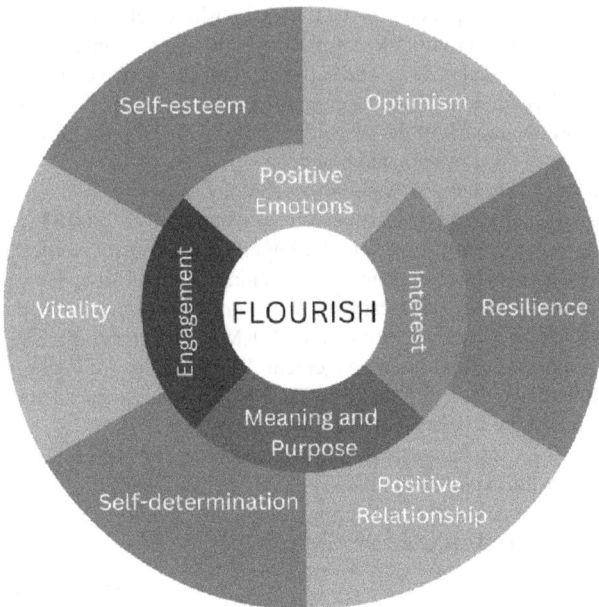

Figure 2.2 Flourishing in Europe model (adapted from Huppert & So, 2013).

interest, meaning, and purpose) and additional elements (self-esteem, optimism, resilience, vitality, self-determination, and positive relationship). For individuals to experience psychological flourishing (optimal wellbeing), they must score highly in all core elements and at least three additional elements (Figure 2.2).

According to the mental health continuum (MHC) model of wellbeing, flourishing is defined as the highest level of emotional, social, and psychological functioning (Keyes, 2002) – it exists along a continuum, with mental disorder on one side, followed by languishing, moderate mental health and flourishing (Figure 2.3). The MHC comprises two main theories of wellbeing: (1) psychological wellbeing (Roepke et al., 2014, 2014) and (2) SWB (Diener, 1984, 2012), as well as an additional model of social wellbeing (Keyes, 1998). The model was developed in response to the World Health Organization's definition of health as a complete mental and social wellbeing, not the absence of disease or infirmity. While a lot was known about what it means to have disease or infirmity, little was known about having complete mental and social wellbeing. Thus, the model was developed to address this gap.

Only a minority of individuals experience flourishing despite widespread reports of happiness (Huppert & So, 2013; Keyes, 2002, p. 2020). Flourishing protects against mood disorders and further symptom development (Burns

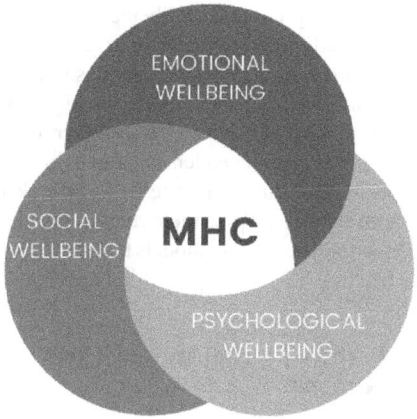

Figure 2.3 Mental health continuum (MHC) model (adapted from Keyes, 2002).

et al., 2022; Schotanus-Dijkstra et al., 2019). The risk of a major depressive episode is ten times more likely among languishers and seven times more likely among moderately well than flourishers (Keyes, 2002). Flourishing is fluid; over a decade, 50% of flourishers experienced a decline in wellbeing (Keyes et al., 2010). Those whose wellbeing declined to moderate levels were seven times more likely to be diagnosed with depression two years later (Keyes et al., 2020). At the same time, most languishers improved their wellbeing over a decade. One crucial reason healthcare professionals need to focus on helping people flourish is the emotional, psychological, and social resources they gain through the process, including buffering, coping with and growing from the effects of trauma (Tedeschi et al., 2018). This can help shift populations' health toward flourishing and reduce the prevalence of mental health issues.

This is why flourishing models can be used as part of the patients' care, and this book will explore the PERMA model as the basis for positive psychology application across the six pillars of lifestyle medicine.

While most positive psychology research applications center around PPIs and learning about the models of wellbeing, recently, researchers identified a missing link in wellbeing literacy. Wellbeing literacy is "a capability to comprehend and compose wellbeing language, across contexts, to use such language to maintain or improve the wellbeing of oneself, others or the world" (Niemiec & Pearce, 2021). As such, how we communicate our wellbeing impacts how we experience it. It comprises six elements (Hou et al., 2021). Individuals are required to have the vocabulary to engage with others about wellbeing. That vocabulary comes from the knowledge we gain by watching videos, attending wellbeing workshops, or reading books such as the book we are currently reading. We also need to have wellbeing skills, which are the specific actions we take to improve our wellbeing, and we need to comprehend the information we read about wellbeing to give us the impact required. When all these elements are present, we can make positive life changes.

Lifestyle medicine and medical care more broadly can harness these models of wellbeing to guide clinical practice and interventions for optimal outcomes. As we've seen the interdependent relationship of these fields propels wellbeing and positive health. In this text, we'll look at how to fully promote wellbeing with the six pillars, their reinforcing link with positive psychology, and the emerging healthcare models that leverage them to achieve and support positive health.

Main Concepts in Positive Psychology and Their Role in Wellbeing Interventions

In this section, we will take a swift journey around the main concepts of positive psychology.

Character Strengths

The taxonomy of character strengths was one of the first endeavors in positive psychology. It was created in response to the deficit-based conceptualization of wellbeing in psychological research, and as such, it has acted as anti-DSM (Diagnostic and Statistical Manual of Mental Disorders). It comprises 6 virtues and 24 character strengths (Pawelski, 2020). See Table 2.1 for details.

The application of character strengths extends from practicing them regularly (e.g. applying strengths when exercising), through to exploring the strengths beneficial to specific aspects of our lives (e.g. using the appreciation of beauty and excellence when going to the local park for a walk), or developing specific strengths to improve our outcomes (e.g. developing self-regulation to lose weight). Given that using strengths is intrinsically rewarding, we are at our best when applying them (Niemiec & Pearce, 2021). This is why, combining

Table 2.1 Values in action (VIA) character strengths

Virtue	Character strength
Wisdom & Knowledge	Love of learning, Perspective, Judgement, Creativity, Curiosity
Humanity	Love, Kindness, Social Intelligence
Justice	Teamwork, Leadership, Fairness
Temperance	Humility, Prudence, Forgiveness, Self-regulation
Transcendence	Appreciation of beauty and excellence, Spirituality, Gratitude, Humour, Hope
Courage	Zest, Bravery, Honesty, Perseverance

Pawelski (2020).

strengths with activities that we do not enjoy can be highly beneficial for finding the motivation to engage with them. These may include regular taking of medication, reducing substance intake, or lonely people connecting with others. Developing character strengths can help us improve our health. For example, a longitudinal study with almost 10,000 older adults showed that over four years, the strength of honesty/integrity was associated with 18% lower risk of lung disease, 11% lower risk of depression, and improved mobility (Taylor & Armor, 1996). In a study with young people, the strength of love of learning was associated with abstinence from drug use (Lyubomirsky et al., 2005). Also, following open-heart surgery, the character strengths of 481 patients were analyzed (Ai et al., 2021). Those who have developed the strength of hope and spirituality before their operation function better in their daily lives after the surgery. Finally, the strength of zest supported patients with pain management (Graziosi et al., 2020).

Similarly, studies with healthcare professionals showed that using specific strengths improved their wellbeing and coping outcomes. For example, hospital physicians who have developed the strengths of hope and zest were less likely to experience emotional exhaustion, whereas humility predicted the physician's wellbeing (Kachel et al., 2021). Thus, with the knowledge of the impact of specific strengths, interventions can be developed to support patients and healthcare professionals.

Whilst we can target the development of specific strengths to help patients and healthcare professionals, research indicates that *any* use of strengths can be beneficial. For example, a systematic review of strength-based interventions for patients with chronic disease showed that they improved their self-efficacy and self-esteem and reduced their depression (Weziak-Bialowolska et al., 2021). In healthcare professionals, using character strengths at work was associated with higher levels of autonomy (Sharot, 2011) and improved the socio-moral climate at work (Höge et al., 2019).

Throughout the book, we will revisit character strengths that support the six pillars of lifestyle medicine. However, it is essential to note that the values in action (VIA) character strengths can be replaced with any strengths. Other strength models exist, such as Strengths Finder or Strengths Profile (Burke & Passmore, 2019). These models provide individuals with the vocabulary they need to express their strengths. However, if they know their strengths and can articulate them well, there is no need to use any models to experience the same positive outcomes.

Hope and Optimism

Optimism is a belief that everything will work out well in the future. It is one of the most misunderstood concepts in psychology, as it is often misinterpreted as wishful thinking. However, the more we delve into the optimism research, the more we realize that it has nothing to do with unrealistic thinking and a lot to do with healthy and adaptive behavior. From the evolutionary perspective, optimism is required for people not to give up (Heifetz & Spiegel, 2000). It fuels persistence and is a foundation for health and wellbeing. When pessimistic, we find it difficult to keep going.

The adaptive role of optimism has emerged in health psychology, following from the research with cancer patients many of whom needed positive illusions to cope (Taylor & Armor, 1996). When faced with trauma, they assumed a positive illusion that it would all work out well for them, even though they were able to control very little of what was happening to them. They needed this, however, to keep going. Optimism is not something that only a few people practice. Neuropsychological research shows that over 70% of people are optimistic (Sheldon & Lyubomirsky, 2021). It is therefore a natural state of mind that helps us survive.

Two psychological theories explain optimism and its benefits. Dispositional optimism views it as a trait, thus it recognizes that some people are predisposed to it. Explanatory style, however, perceives it as a thinking style and acknowledges that everyone can learn to think more optimistically regardless of their personality or hereditary inclinations (Schiavon et al., 2017). As such, when a bad thing happens to people, they may react to it in a pessimistic or optimistic way. If we tend to steer toward pessimism, to change this, we need to change our thinking and the benefits of optimism will follow. The three questions we need to ask ourselves are:

1 Who is responsible for this?

When bad things happen, pessimists take full responsibility for the events without considering the circumstances. However, often, if not always, circumstances play an important role in adverse outcomes. Optimists consider those circumstances, which allows them to move past self-blame and toward resolving an issue.

For example, Margo had an epileptic seizure for the first time in ten years. If she were a pessimist, she would blame herself for the "stupidity of going to a nightclub with flashing lights last night." If she were an optimist, she would consider the situation's circumstances. It was the 20th anniversary of her marriage, a special night. Given the years of being free from the epileptic seizures and the doctor's green light for her to drive and live her life to the full, she thought it was safe. Thus, an optimistic Margo would find a way to consider the circumstances associated with her decision, and as such, she would not self-blame. A pessimistic Margo would spend much time self-blaming and perhaps not taking action to resolve the issue.

2 How long will it last?

Pessimists tend to catastrophize. So, when they experience bad events, they may think bad things will last forever. Optimists, on the other hand, believe that bad things are temporary. They are, therefore, more likely to believe that the good times will come back soon. This gives them the hope to keep going, even in the worst circumstances.

For example, Michael has tried hard to get into an exercise routine. He kept it up for a few months, but then he became busy at work, and his practice became less frequent until he stopped going to the gym altogether. He was there before, started exercising regularly, and gave up. If he were a pessimist, he would just become frustrated about himself, saying: "Some things never change. I will always quit, no matter how well I did before." If he were an optimist, he would focus on the temporality of this situation. "I quit it now, but I will get back there again, just like I did before."

3   What aspects of my life does it impact?

Pessimists tend to see a bad event as a chain reaction. When they experience adverse situations, they tend to see it as the first of many bad things happening to them. Optimists, however, are better at compartmentalizing their lives. They isolate the bad situation in the context of all the good things that happen to them.

For example, Kate had an injury that prevented her from going for daily walks. If she were a pessimist she would say: "By the time my injury heals, I'll become fat, unfit, and depressed." If she were an optimist she would say: "Fine, I have an injury and I can't go for a walk. At least I have good family and friends who will visit me and keep me sane."

Hope differs from optimism as it incorporates a plan for making changes (Carver & Scheier, 2003). When hopeful, we not only have a will to keep going, but also a pathway for making it happen. As such, optimism is not just a wishful thinking, it is a strategy for helping patients feel in control.

A systematic review of the literature relating to health and optimism showed that both concepts were associated with each other (Peterson & Seligman, 2004). Optimism was associated with lower mortality rates, improved immune function, better cardiovascular outcomes, cancer outcomes, pregnancy outcomes, pain management, to mention a few. Furthermore, optimists were more likely to eat better quality food (Ait-Hadad et al., 2020) and sleep (Hernandez et al., 2020). Also, optimism and hope are important ingredients in managing chronic disease as they are associated with healthier behaviors regardless of individuals' health status (Ryff, 2014). At the same time, unrealistic optimism was associated with higher risk of lung cancer relating to smoking (Dillard et al., 2006), thus a balanced approach is required to practicing optimism.

Positive Emotions

For decades, researchers undermined the importance of positive emotions. In one of the primary theories of emotions, Paul Ekman (2004) identified six core emotions based on facial expressions, such as fear, anger, disgust, sadness, happiness, and surprise, with most leaning toward the negative. Negative emotions were deemed crucial for evolutionary purposes, serving as warnings against potential dangers. Conversely, positive emotions were often overlooked in empirical enquiries, as they seemed to contribute little beyond fostering happiness. This perception shifted when researchers like Alice Isen from Cornell University conducted experiments demonstrating the vital role of positive emotions in our lives (Moskowitz & Saslow, 2014). Isen's findings revealed that positive emotions facilitate creativity, problem-solving, decision-making, and negotiation, forming the basis for the Broaden-and-build theory, which posits that positive emotions expand our minds and construct psychological, intellectual, and social resources for thriving (Fredrickson, 2001).

Now, the broaden-and-build theory stands as the predominant explanation for the role of positive emotions in our psyche. When we guide students in generating positive emotions (Fredrickson and Joiner, 2018), they undergo a temporary broadening of ideas, enabling them to devise more creative solutions and perceive previously unseen perspectives. Establishing a habit of inducing and regularly experiencing positive emotions serves as a protective shield against pathologies. Positive emotions initiate a transformative upward spiral that fosters continual growth in the future. Consequently, patients who have frequently experienced positive emotions before a crisis find that, rather than diminishing during the crisis, their positivity amplifies, with emotions like hope significantly contributing to the development of resilience and wellbeing (Fredrickson et al., 2003). These insights underscore the usefulness of assisting patients in accessing and further developing their positive emotions.

While positive emotions are transitory, their full experience sets off a cascade of processes that enhance long-term wellbeing (Fredrickson and Joiner, 2002). They positively impact physical health (Kok et al., 2013), alleviate illness symptoms, enhance life purpose, and encourage seeking social support over isolation (Fredrickson et al., 2008). Crucially, positive emotions substantially contribute to psychological flourishing (Kahneman & Riis., 2005) and play a pivotal role in transforming the negative emotions' vicious cycle into a beneficial cycle that reduces suicidal thoughts (Joiner, 2005), depression, anxiety (Garland et al., 2010), and self-harm (Morris et al., 2014). Thus, positive emotions not only exist to bring happiness but, despite their fleeting nature, also act as a safeguard against experiencing ill-being.

Meaning in Life

Meaning *in* life differs from the meaning *of* life, which questions our existence. Within positive psychology, we explore the meaning in life, which is perceived as the consistency in which individuals understand themselves, in the context of their life and how they plan to live their meaning by having a clear life purpose (Steger et al., 2015). As such, meaning in life is about knowing who we are, why we are here, what is important to us, what we are hoping to achieve, and comprehending how our life experiences have shaped us into the people we are today. While *meaning* refers to the theoretical aspect of our experience, *purpose* is the application of it.

Understanding our meaning in life is beneficial to us, nonetheless, the search for meaning is linked with a range of adverse mental health outcomes (Li et al., 2021). When individuals have a clarity about their life meaning, they are more likely to report improved physical health (Roepke et al., 2014), experience less pathologies, such as depression, and show higher levels of psychological and emotional wellbeing (Steger, 2017). Most importantly, however, meaning offers mental health protection during testing times (Wong, 2011), more so than experiencing positive emotions or any other types of wellbeing components. It helps us make sense of our suffering, be it a chronic disease or other diagnosis.

Lower levels of meaning in life are predictive of daily smoking (Steger, 2017). Furthermore, four-year longitudinal research showed that smokers' life meaning has decreased during this time (Thege et al., 2013). This effect extends beyond tobacco, as presence of life meaning is strongly associated with using less substances such as alcohol and drugs (Csabonyi & Phillips, 2020). Thus, the impact of substances can have detrimental effect on eudaimonic wellbeing.

Conclusion

Character strengths, hope, optimism, other positive emotions, and meaning in life represent key constructs in positive psychology. Interventions for wellbeing are built on these constructs and can be applied to promote or support emotional as well as physical wellbeing with relevance to medical practice. In the next several chapters, we'll take a look at the science and practice – including case studies of typical or amalgamated patients – of how such interventions interlink with lifestyle medicine pillars.

References

Ai, A. L., Fincham, F. D., & Carretta, H. (2021). ADL and IADL following open-heart surgery: The role of a character strength factor and preoperative medical comorbidities. *Journal of Religion and Health.* https://doi.org/10.1007/s10943-020-01146-w.

Ait-Hadad, W., Bénard, M., Shankland, R., Kesse-Guyot, E., Robert, M., Touvier, M., Hercberg, S., Buscail, C., & Péneau, S. (2020). Optimism is associated with diet quality, food group consumption and snacking behavior in a general population. *Nutrition Journal, 19*(1), 6. https://doi.org/10.1186/s12937-020-0522-7.

Burns, R. A., Windsor, T., Butterworth, P., & Anstey, K. J. (2022). The protective effects of wellbeing and flourishing on long-term mental health risk. *SSM- Mental Health,* 2.100052. https://doi.org/10.1016/j.ssmmh.2021.100052

Burke, J., & Dunne, P. J. (2022). Lifestyle medicine pillars as predictors of psychological flourishing. *Frontiers in Psychology*, 13, 963806. https://doi.org/10.3389/fpsyg.2022.963806

Burke, J., Dunne, P. J., Meehan, T., O'Boyle, C., & van Nieuwerburgh, C. (2023a). *Positive health, 100+ research-based positive psychology and lifestyle medicine tools to enhance your wellbeing.* Rutledge.

Burke, J., Dunne, P., & Byrne, E. (2023b). Positive health interventions: An emerging concept. In J. Burke, I. Boniwell, B. Frates, L. Lianov, & C.A. O'Boyle (Eds.), *The Routledge International handbook of positive health* (pp. 191–207). Routledge.

Burke, J., & Passmore, J. (2019). Strengths based coaching: A positive psychology intervention. In L. E. Van Zyl, & S. Rothmann Sr (Eds.), *Theoretical approaches to multi-cultural positive psychological interventions* (pp. 463–476). Springer.

Carver, C. S. & Scheier, M. (2003). Optimism. In Lopez, S. J. & Snyder, C. R. *Positive psychological assessment: A handbook of models and measures (pp. 75–89).* American Psychological Association. https://doi.org/10.1037/10612-005.

Csabonyi, M. & Phillips, L. J. (2020). Meaning in life and substance use. *Journal of Humanistic Psychology*. 60(2), 3–19. https://doi.org/10.1177/0022167816687674

Diener, E. (1984). Subjective well-being. *Psychological Bulletin*, *95*(3), 542–575. https://doi.org//10.1037/0033-2909.95.3.542.

Diener, E. (2012). New findings and future directions for subjective well-being research. *American Psychologist*, *67*(8), 590–597. https://doi.org/10.1037/a0029541.

Diener, E., Pressman, S. D., Hunter, J., & Delgadillo-Chase, D. (2017). If, why, and when subjective well-being influences health, and future needed research. *Applied Psychology. Health and Well-Being*, *9*(2), 133–167. https://doi.org/10.1037/a0029541.

Dillard, A. J., McCaul, K. D., & Klein, W. M. (2006). Unrealistic optimism in smokers: Implications for smoking myth endorsement and self-protective motivation. *Journal of Health Communication*, *11*(Suppl 1), 93–102. https://doi.org/10.1080/10810730600637343.

Ekman, P. (2004). What we become emotional about. In A.S.R. Manstead, N. Frijda, A. Fischer (Eds.), *Feelings and emotions* (pp. 119–135). Cambridge University Press. https://doi.org/10.1017/CBO9780511806582.008

Fletcher, G. (2016). *The philosophy of well-being: An introduction.* Routledge.

Fredrickson, B., Cohn, M., Coffey, K. A., Pek, J., & Fonkel, S.(2008), Open hearts build lives: Positive emotions, induced loving-kindness meditation, build consequential personal resources. *Journal of Personality and Social Psychology*, *95*(5):1045–1062. https://doi.org/10.1037/a0013262

Fredrickson, B. L. (2001). The role of positive emotions in positive psychology: The broaden-and-build theory of positive emotions. *American Psychologist*, *56*(3), 218–226. https://doi.org/10.1037/0003-066X.56.3.218.

Fredrickson, B. L., & Joiner, T. (2002). Positive emotions trigger upward spirals toward emotional well-being. *Psychological Science*, 13(2). https://doi.org/10.1111/1467-9280.00431

Fredrickson, B. L., & Joiner, T. (2018). Reflections on positive emotions and upward spirals. *Perspectives on Psychological Science*, 13(2). https://doi.org/10.1177/1745691617692106

Fredrickson, B. L., Tugade, M. M., Waugh, C. E., & Larkin, G. R. (2003). What good are emotions in crises? A prospective study of resilience and emotions following the terrorist attacks on the United States September 11th, 2001. *Journal of Personality and Social Psychology, 84*(2), 365–376.

Garland, E. L., Fredrickson, B., Kring, A. M., Johnson, D. P., Meyer, P. S., & Penn, D. L. (2010). Upward spirals of positive emotions counter downward spirals of negativity: Insights from the broaden-and-build theory and affective neuroscience on the treatment of emotion dysfunctions and deficits in psychopathology. *Clinical Psychology Review, 30*(7), 849–64. https://doi.org/10.1016/j.cpr.2010.03.002.

Grand View Research. (2023). *Global Personal Development Market.*

Graziosi, M., Yaden, D., Clifton, J., Mikanik, N., & Niemiec, R. M. (2022). A strengths-based approach to chronic pain. *Journal of Positive Psychology, 17*(3), 400–408. https://doi.org/10.1080/17439760.2020.1858337.

Heifetz, A., & Spiegel, Y. (2000). *On the evolutionary emergence of optimism. SSRN.*

Hernandez, R., Vu, T. T., Kershaw, K. N., Boehm, J. K., Kubzansky, L. D., Carnethon, M., Trudel-Fitzgerald, C., Knutson, K. L., Colangelo, L. A., & Liu, K. (2020). The association of optimism with sleep duration and quality: Findings from the coronary artery risk and development in young adults (CARDIA) study. *Behavioral Medicine (Washington, D.C.), 46*(2), 100–111. https://doi.org/10.1080/08964289.2019.1575179.

Höge, T., Strecker, C., Hausler, M., Huber, A., & Höfer, S. (2019). Perceived socio-moral climate and the applicability of signature character strengths at work: A study among hospital physicians. *Applied Research in Quality of Life.* https://doi.org/10.1007/s11482-018-9697-x.

Hou, H., Chin, T. C., Slemp, G. R., & Oades, L. G. (2021). Wellbeing literacy: Conceptualization, measurement, and preliminary empirical findings from students, parents and school staff. *International Journal of Environmental Research and Public Health, 18*(4), 1485. https://doi.org/10.3390/ijerph18041485.

Huppert, F. A., & So, T. T. (2013). Flourishing across europe: Application of a new conceptual framework for defining well-being. *Social Indicators, 110*(3), 837–861. https://doi.org/10.1007/s11205-011-9966-7.

Joiner, T. (2005). *Why people die by suicide.* Harvard University Press.

Kachel, T., Huber, A., Strecker, C., Hoge, T., & Hofer, S. (2021). Reality meets belief: A mixed methods study on character strengths and well-being of hospital physicians. *Frontiers in Psychology, 12.* https://doi.org/10.3389/fpsyg.2021.547773

Kahneman, D., & Riis, J. (2005). Living, and thinking about it: Two perspectives on life. In F. A. Huppert, N. Baylis, & B. Keverne (Eds.), *The science of wellbeing* (pp. 285–304). Oxford University Press. https://doi.org/10.1093/acprof:oso/9780198567523.003.0011

Keyes, C. L. M. (1998). Social well-being. *Social Psychology Quarterly, 61*(2), 121–140. https://doi.org/10.2307/2787065.

Keyes, C. L. M. (2002). The mental health continuum: From languishing to flourishing. *Journal of Health and Social Research, 43*, 207–222. https://doi.org/10.2307/3090197

Keyes, C. L. M., Dhingra, S. S., & Simoes, E. J. (2010). Change in level of positive mental health as a predictor of future risk of mental illness. *American Journal of Public Health, 100*(12), 2366–2371. https://doi.org/10.2105/AJPH.2010.192245.

Keyes, C. L. M., Yao, J., Hybels, C. F., Milstein, G., & Proeschold-Bell, R. J. (2020). Are changes in positive mental health associated with increased likelihood of depression over a two year period? A test of the mental health promotion and protection hypotheses. *Journal of Affective Disorders, 270,* 136–142. https://doi.org/10.1007/s11482-018-9697-x

Kok, B. E., Coffey, K. A., Cohn, M. A., Catalina, L. I., Vacharkulksemsuk, T., Algoe, S., Brantley, M., & Fredrickson, B. L. (2013). How positive emotions build physical health: Perceived social connections account for the upward spiral between positive emotions and vagal tone. *Psychological Science, 27*(4), 1123–32. https://doi.org/10.1177/0956797612470827.

Layous, K., Hyunjung, L., Incheol, C., & Lyubomirsky, S. (2013). Culture matters when designing a successful happiness-increasing activity: A comparison of the United States and South korea. *Journal of Cross-Cultural Psychology, 44*(8), 1294–1303. https://doi.org/10.1177/0022022113487591.

Li, J.-B., Dou, K., & Liang, Y. (2021). The relationship between presence of meaning, search for meaning, and subjective well-being: A three-level meta-analysis based on the meaning in life questionnaire. *Journal of Happiness Studies: An Interdisciplinary Forum on Subjective Well-Being, 22,* 467–489. https://doi.org/10.1007/s10902-020-00230-y

Lyubomirsky, S., & Layous, K. (2013). How do simple positive activities increase well-being? *Current Directions in Psychological Science, 22*(1), 57–62. https://doi.org/10.1177/0963721412469809.

Lyubomirsky, S., Sheldon, K. M., & Schkade, D. (2005). Pursuing happiness: The architecture of sustainable change. *Review of General Psychology, 9*(2), 111–131. https://doi.org/10.1037/1089-2680.9.2.111.

Ma, M., Kibler, J. L., Dollar, K. M., Sly, K., Samuels, D., Benford, M. W., Coleman, M., Lott, L., Patterson, K., & Wiley, F. (2008). The relationship of character strengths to sexual behaviors and related risks among African American adolescents. *International Journal of Behavioral Medicine, 15*(4), 319–327. https://doi.org/10.1080/10705500802365573.

Morris, C., Simpson, J., Simpson, M., & Beesley, F. (2014). Cultivating positive emotions: A useful adjunct when working with people who self-harm? *Clinical Psychology & Psychotherapy, 21*(4), 352–362. https://doi.org/10.1002/cpp.1836.

Moskowitz, J. T. & Saslow, L. R. (2014). Health and psychology: The importance of positive affect. In Tugade, M. M., N., Shiota, M. N., & L. & Kirby, L. D. (Eds.), *Handbook of positive emotions* (pp. 413–431). https://doi.org/10.1093/acprof:oso/9780199926725.001.0001.

Niemiec, R. M., & Pearce, R. (2021). The practice of character strengths: Unifying definitions, principles, and exploration of What's soaring, emerging, and ripe with potential in science and in practice. *Frontiers in Psychology, 11,* 590220. https://doi.org/10.3390/ijerph18020719

Oades, L. G., Jarden, A., Hou, H., Ozturk, C., Williams, P., Slemp, G. R., & Huang, L. (2021). Wellbeing literacy: A capability model for wellbeing science and practice. *International Journal of Environmental Research and Public Health, 18*(2), 719. https://doi.org/10.3390/ijerph18020719.

Parks, A., & Biswas Diener, R. (2013). Positive interventions: Past, present, and future. In T. B. Kashdan, & J. Ciarrochi (Eds.), *Mindfulness, acceptance, and positive psychology: The even foundations of well-being* (pp. 140–165). New Harbinger Publications, Inc.

Pawelski, J. O. (2020). The elements model: Toward a new generation of positive psychology interventions. *Journal of Positive Psychology, 15*(5), 675–679. https://doi.org/10.1080/17439760.2020.1789710.

Peterson, C., & Seligman, M. E. P. (2004). *Character strengths and virtues: A handbook and classification.* Oxford University Press; American Psychological Association. https://doi.org/10.1080/17439760.2013.777766

Rasmussen, H. N., Scheier, M. F., & Greenhouse, J. B. (2009). Optimism and physical health: A meta-analytic review. *Annals of Behavioral Medicine: a Publication of the Society of Behavioral Medicine, 37*(3), 239–256. https://doi.org/10.1007/s12160-009-9111-x.

Roepke, A. M., Jayawickreme, E., & Riffle, O. M. (2014). Meaning and health: A systematic review. *Applied Research in Quality of Life, 9,* 1055–1079.

Ryff, C. D. (1989). Happiness is everything, or is it? Explorations on the meaning of psychological well-being. *Journal of Personality and Social Psychology, 57*(6), 1069–1081. https://doi.org/10.1037/0022-3514.57.6.1069.

Ryff, C. D. (2014). Psychological well-being revisited: Advances in the science and practice of eudaimonia. *Psychotherapy and Psychosomatics, 83*(1), 10–28. https://doi.org/10.1159/000353263.

Schiavon, C. C., Marchetti, E., Gurgel, L. G., Busnello, F. M., & Reppold, C. T. (2017). Optimism and hope in chronic disease: A systematic review. *Frontiers in Psychology, 7,* 2022. https://doi.org/10.3389/fpsyg.2016.02022

Schotanus-Dijkstra, M., Keyes, C., de Graaf, R., & ten Have, M. (2019). Recovery from mood and anxiety disorders: The influence of positive mental health. *Journal of Affective Disorders, 252,* 107–113. https://doi.org/10.1016/j.jad.2019.04.051

Seligman, M. E. P. (1986). Explanatory style as a predictor of productivity and quitting among life insurance sales agents. *Journal of Personality and Social Psychology, 50*(4), 832–836. https://doi.org/10.1037/0022-3514.50.4.832.

Seligman, M. E. P., & Csikszentmihalyi, M. (2000). Positive psychology: An introduction. *American Psychologist, 55*(1), 5–14. https://doi.org/10.1037/0003-066X.55.1.5.

Seligman, M. E. P. (2002). *Authentic happiness: Using the new positive psychology to realize your potential for lasting fulfillment.* Free Press.

Seligman, M. E. P. (2011). *Flourish: A visionary new understanding of happiness and well-being.* Atria.

Seligman, M. E. P., & Csikszentmihalyi, M. (2000). Positive psychology: An introduction. *American Psychologist.* 55(1), 5–14. https://doi.org/10.1037/0003-066X.55.1.5

Sharot, T. (2011). The optimism bias. *Current Biology, 21*(23). https://doi.org/10.1016/j.cub.2011.10.030

Sheldon, K. M., & Lyubomirsky, S. (2021). Revisiting the sustainable happiness model and pie chart: Can happiness be successfully pursued? *The Journal of Positive Psychology, 16*(2), 145–154. https://doi.org/10.1080/17439760.2019.1689421.

Steger, M., Fitch-Martin, A., Donnelly, J., & Rickard, K. (2015). Meaning in life and health: proactive health orientation links meaning in life to health variables among American undergraduates. *Journal of Happiness Studies, 16,* 583–597. https://doi.org/10.1007/s10902-014-9523-6

Steger, M. F. (2017). Meaning in life and wellbeing. In: Slade, M., Oades, L. & Jarden, A. (Eds.), *Wellbeing, recovery and mental health* (pp. 75–85). Cambridge University Press.

Strecker, C., Huber, A., Höge, T., Hausler, M., & Höfer, S. (2019). Identifying thriving workplaces in hospitals: Work characteristics and the applicability of character strengths at work. *Applied Research in Quality of Life.* https://doi.org/10.1007/s11482-018-9693-1.

Taylor, S. E., & Armor, D. A. (1996). Positive illusions and coping with adversity. *Journal of Personality, 64*(4), 873–898. https://doi.org/10.1111/j.1467-6494.1996. tb00947.x.

Tedeschi R. G., Shakespeare-Finch, J., Taku, K., & Calhoun, L. G. (2018) *Posttraumatic growth, theory, research, and applications.* Rutledge.

Thege, B. K., Bachner, Y. G., Martos, T., & Kushnir, T. (2009). Meaning in life: Does it play a role in smoking? *Substance Use & Misuse, 44*(11), 1566–1577. https://doi. org/10.1080/10826080802495096.

Thege, B. K., Urbán, R., & Kopp, M. S. (2013). Four-year prospective evaluation of the relationship between meaning in life and smoking status. *Substance Abuse Treatment, Prevention, and Policy, 8*, 8. https://doi.org/10.1186/1747-597X-8-8

Weziak-Bialowolska, D., Bialowolski, P., & Niemiec, R. M. (2021). Being good, doing good: The role of honesty and integrity for health. *Social Science and Medicine, 291.* https://doi.org/10.1016/j.socscimed.2021.114494

Wong, P. (2011). Reclaiming positive psychology: A meaning-centered approach to sustainable growth and radical empiricism. *Journal of Humanistic Psychology, 51*(4). https://doi.org/10.1016/j.socscimed.2021.114494

Yan, T., Chan, C. W. H., Chow, K. M., Zheng, W., & Sun, M. (2020). A systematic review of the effects of character strengths-based intervention on the psychological well-being of patients suffering from chronic illnesses. *Journal of Advanced Nursing, 76*(7), 1567–1580. https://doi.org/10.1111/jan.14356

3   Positive Psychology and Healthy Eating for Positive Health

Chapter Overview

This chapter provides a brief overview of the science and introduces practical clinical coaching applications of the PERMA framework and other positive psychology techniques to promote healthy eating and using healthy eating to improve emotional wellbeing for achieving positive health. The reciprocal, reinforcing link between healthy eating and positive emotions is emphasized.

Introduction

Positive emotions and healthy eating, like other healthy behaviors, have a reciprocal, reinforcing relationship. That is, positive emotions can drive healthy eating and, inversely, healthy eating increases positive emotions. This link, along with an increase in supportive vantage resources that are developed, leads to an upward and outward spiral of lifestyle change. As a result, the change may be achievable and sustainable (Van Cappellen et al., 2018).

An unhealthy lifestyle has consequences beyond health. For example, the impact of excess food on overweight and obese children extends to an increased risk of bullying, depression, and poor social integration (Puhl & Latner, 2007). Similarly, overweight adults experience lower levels of confidence, are less likely to join in social interactions and report lower levels of psychological wellbeing (Magallares & Pais-Ribeiro, 2014). Thus, the issues caused by poor eating habits extend beyond health and into psychology.

Recently, a concept of food wellbeing was introduced and defined as "a positive psychological, physical, emotional, and social relationship with food at both the individual and societal levels" (Block et al., 2011, p. 6). It refers to the impact of eating well on psycho-social wellbeing for both individuals

DOI: 10.4324/9781003428909-3

and groups and shifts a focus from food as a source of health to food as a source of wellbeing. However, the link between food and wellbeing needs to be further investigated, because the exact link remains unclear (Holden, 2019). According to some reports, food is a source of happiness and increased wellbeing (e.g. Lesani et al., 2016; Mujcic & Oswald, 2016; Warner et al., 2017).

A Plant-Predominant Eating Pattern Increases Positive Affect

A healthy eating pattern consisting of mostly plant-based whole foods offers many benefits for health and wellbeing (Frates et al., 2020; Sarin et al., 2022). Specifically, vegetable and fruit consumption is associated with increases in positive affect and happiness (Fararouei et al., 2013; Mujcic & Oswald, 2016; White et al., 2013). According to one study, at least 7–8 servings of fruit or vegetables per day are needed to see meaningful changes (Mujcic & Oswald, 2016). These changes include feeling calmer, happier, and more energetic than normal; and the positive mood can last into the next day.

In a study with over 13,000 participants in the UK, the researchers found that participants' mental wellbeing decreased with each portion decrease in vegetable and fruit consumption (Stranges et al., 2014). However, the relationship of obesity, lower vegetable and fruit consumption, and poor mental wellbeing is not fully delineated.

The situation becomes even more complex when we analyze the results of psychological flourishing. Mental health includes the absence of depression and anxiety. Psychological flourishing incorporates the experiences of wellbeing that protect us against depression and anxiety and help us live a good life. A study that explored psychological flourishing, happiness, and life satisfaction among over 80,000 participants showed that eating five servings of fruit and vegetables a day was not enough to experience the highest levels of flourishing (Blanchflower et al., 2013). At five servings a day, individuals' wellbeing plateaued. Instead, eating seven portions of fruit and vegetables daily was associated with the highest psychological wellbeing, satisfaction, and happiness.

Similarly, New Zealand research with 9,514 participants showed that individuals who consumed sugary drinks 5–6 times a week (as well as lived a sedentary life and reported restless sleep) reported lower levels of psychological flourishing measured through a range of flourishing scales assessing such elements of wellbeing as their experiences of positive emotions, optimism, self-esteem, engagement, etc. (Prendergast et al., 2016). Interestingly, the study showed that 43% of New Zealanders regularly consume sugary drinks, and only 25% had a regular fruit and vegetable intake. Nevertheless, the highest levels of wellbeing were noted among those who consume fruit and vegetables. Again, this study identified a correlation between that behavior and wellbeing but did not determine whether consuming fruit and vegetables as an intervention results in higher levels of subjective wellbeing. A study with 541 medical students delved deeper into fruit and vegetable intake and nutritional habits (Lesani et al., 2016). It showed that those who reported the highest levels of happiness consumed more than eight portions of fruit and vegetables a day. They also had three meals (including breakfast) a day and 1–2 snacks. This increase may be due to increased positive emotions individuals experience when eating fruit and vegetables. A study with over a thousand participants showed that positive affect increased systematically with almost every portion of fruit and vegetables (Warner et al., 2017). The highest positive emotions were recorded for individuals who ate more than eight fruits and veg but did not increase at levels above that amount.

Apart from positive emotions and happiness, healthy eating can also improve individuals' eudaimonic wellbeing, curiosity, and creativity (Conner & Silvia, 2015), thus it impacts them on a cognitive, not only emotional level. In this study, participants were asked to complete an internet diary for 13 consecutive days. Research showed that those who ate more fruit and vegetables as opposed to sweets and chips reported significantly higher levels of psychological flourishing associated with being more engaged in life, seeing life as more purposeful and meaningful, and having higher levels of optimism for the future. All these outcomes are therefore related to the choice of healthy and unhealthy food participants ate.

However, the more surprising findings in this study showed that fruit and vegetable consumption made people more curious and creative about engaging with their own thoughts and the world around them. Curiosity is a unique quality that young children tend to experience frequently and as they progress through their education the capacity for experiencing curiosity declines. Yet, curiosity among adults is associated with higher levels of various aspects of wellbeing (Kashdan, 2009). Curiosity facilitates psychological growth and connection with people.

While not all aspects of curiosity are helpful for wellbeing, curiosity moderates our mood. For example, in a study that asked participants to use a diary of moods for 21 days, the researchers found that when individuals reported higher levels of flourishing, their stressor-related negative mood was higher (Drake et al., 2022). Interestingly, however, on days when they displayed lower levels of curiosity, their mood declined. Thus, curiosity during the day acts as a protective mechanism for enhancing our mood and helping us live a good life. This is why it is exciting to see research showing that eating more portions of fruit and vegetables is associated with higher levels of curiosity (Conner & Silvia, 2015). It is yet another psychological benefit of eating well.

Positive Psychology Techniques Can Support Healthy Eating

Meaning and Healthy Eating

While a healthy eating pattern can increase positive emotions, inversely, being happier is associated with greater fruit and vegetable consumption (Gardner et al., 2014). One explanation offered by researchers is that the perception of the importance of healthy eating to achieve long-term goals is enhanced by positive emotions. Keeping in mind that a range of emotions can enrich one's life, such as eudaimonic experiences, linking meaning to the desired change, can be a powerful behavioral nudge. Studies also reveal that feeling more positively in general can help individuals eat more healthfully (Ait-Hadad et al., 2020; Hingle et al., 2014; Pänkäläinen et al., 2018; Whatnall et al., 2019). The more immediate feelings of wellbeing with a healthy eating pattern reinforce the desire to eat healthy foods (Gardner et al., 2014; Mujcic & Oswald, 2016).

Positive Psychology Interventions (PPIs) for Healthy Eating

By using positive psychology techniques, individuals can learn to appreciate the positive aspects of healthy eating, such as enjoying delicious, nutritious food, and the sense of accomplishment that comes from taking good care of themselves. PPIs can help individuals develop supportive habits and routines related to healthy eating, such as meal planning and preparation with family and friends, and mindful eating. Identifying and applying character strengths and values is another positive psychology method that empowers individuals to eat healthy foods. Examples include the perseverance and optimism to start a new healthy eating action plan after previous unsuccessful attempts and the deep appreciation for the beauty and taste of healthy foods.

Positive Experiences During Meals

It is not only the good food we consume that matters but also how we do it. In an experiment with 1,467 families, individuals were asked to approach family meals differently (Ho et al., 2020). While their objective was to eat a lower-sugar diet, they were asked to do it with their family by introducing positive psychology concepts such as joy, gratitude, and savoring. For example, it involved:

Joy

1   Sharing with their family member a joyful experience of healthy eating
2   Searching for joy in a healthy diet
3   Reminiscing a joyful experience for individuals and their families

Gratitude

4 Appreciating family strengths when embarking on a healthy diet
5 Expressing gratitude, with words (e.g. thank you) or actions (e.g. turning off devices), for the food family eats or the time they spend together at the table

Savoring

6 Savoring the healthy diet
7 Treasuring the time with family while eating good food.

The "fun" activities families were encouraged to practice included:

1 Family members preparing and eating a low-sugar food together
2 Families reading food labels together and identifying the low, medium, and high sugar content
3 Families showing appreciation for the food they ate
4 Families selecting a fruit of their choice as a "gift" to their family members
5 Blindfolding family members and giving them food products, asking them to use their other senses and guess how much sugar each product contained
6 Preparing food and savoring it together, feeling love and care around the table.

This intervention resulted in participants reducing their sugar intake. In addition to the health outcomes, the intervention was also effective in promoting family harmony at one-month follow-up and subjective wellbeing at three months follow-up.

Environment or Setting of the Meals

Many factors impact our food enjoyment (Macht et al., 2005). The type of food we consume impacts our wellbeing differently. The same food can become a positive, neutral, or negative experience for different individuals, depending on their individual preferences. The physical environment of the food we consume also matters. Whether we eat our food in a kitchen, standing up at the island unit, in our favorite coffee shop, or in a fancy restaurant, our experience will differ. All this also depends on our preferences, as for some people eating in a nice restaurant may evoke pleasure, whereas others will report social anxiety. The social factors of our food consumption have a significant impact on our wellbeing too. Consuming food in a company of others is more enjoyable than eating on our own. However, it comes with a challenge of eating too much (Herman, 2017).

Mindset Associated with Healthy Eating

In addition to the environmental setting of food consumption, our mindset impacts wellbeing. For some, food is a physiological process of consuming calories for survival. For others, it is a highly hedonic experience that influences their eating outcomes. As a hedonic experience, food can become a comfort on a bad day. As such, it is used for coping with adversity. It allows individuals to balance out the adverse events of their day with a highly enjoyable food at night. However, just because we eat comforting food doesn't mean it will make us feel good.

To help us amplify this experience of mindset associated with eating, we can use the emotional regulation model (Table 3.1).

Self-Compassion

Self-compassion has long been associated with good health. It is the practice of guarding oneself against suffering or feeling inferior by using compassion inwardly to create a self-kindness response to challenging situations (Neff, 2003). It comprises six dimensions: 1) self-kindness – giving oneself support and understanding, as we would give our friends, 2) self-judgment – avoiding giving oneself harsh judgments, 3) common humanity – realizing that everyone struggles, fails, and makes mistakes 4) isolation – not feeling on your own, connecting with others, avoiding isolation, 5) mindfulness – being mindful of internal processes, aware of our own suffering, and 6) over-identity – avoiding over-identifying self with our negative thoughts and emotions (Philips et al., 2019).

Table 3.1 Emotional regulation model: Examples

Example 1	Example 2
1. Situation selection I will go out with my partner for a dinner	I will cook a new recipe
2. Situation modification We will select our favorite restaurant and ask for a table by the window	I will test this new plant-based recipe that looks delicious in the picture
3. Attentional deployment As we sit at the table, I enjoy every bite and notice the restaurant ambiance	I focus my attention on food preparation and cut my vegetables with more care than usual
4. Cognitive change I choose to take my savoring of food up a level and engage all my senses	I praise my effort after each part of the food prep and allow myself to feel a sense of pride
5. Response modulation I tell my partner how much I am enjoying the night	I tell my family they are up for a real treat this evening

Increasingly evidence suggests that self-compassion plays a vital role in eating disorders (Messer et al., 2021). With this in mind, we have designed a study with middle-aged adults exploring the correlation between intuitive eating and self-compassion (Irmisher et al., forthcoming). In our research, we controlled for wellbeing, as we wanted to ensure that our participants' existing psychological wellness did not influence their outcomes. Intuitive eating is an adaptive method for reducing overeating that relies on hunger and satiety clues. It comprises four components: (1) unconditional permission to eat, (2) eating for physical rather than emotional reasons, (3) reliance on hunger and satiety cues, and (4) body-food choice congruence (Tylka & Kroon van Diest, 2013).

Our research showed that self-compassion predicted participants' intuitive eating and two components of self-compassion played a significant role in helping individuals moderate their food intake. The first component was a lack of self-judgment. When participants consciously avoided thinking harshly of themselves, they were more likely to use intuitive eating as a technique for moderating their food intake. Secondly, common humanity was also associated with improved intuitive eating. This is a realization that we all struggle in life and we all make mistakes and fail every now and then. Also, we all get up and keep doing it again. Given these research findings, it is crucial that healthcare professionals avoid stigma; yet, some show a significant weight bias, which in turn impacts their patients negatively (Phelan et al., 2015). Instead, showing more compassion about weight loss may prove more helpful to patients and enhance their motivation for change (Neff, 2023). The box provides a compassionate activity that physicians can use to improve individuals' wellbeing.

Self-Compassion Journal (Neff, 2023)

Keep a daily journal in which you describe your daily struggles in a supportive, compassionate way. This will help you bring more compassion, common humanity, kindness, and mindfulness into your life.

Changing Your Critical Self-Talk (Neff, 2023)

When you catch yourself speaking harshly about yourself, stop and acknowledge this. Then, try to reframe it in a friendly way. What would your friend say to you?

Neff et al. (2020) have developed a program designed specifically for healthcare professionals to help them increase self-compassion and improve their own wellbeing, in addition to helping patients. It is a six-week, one-day-a-week course that guides them through tips and techniques to build self-compassion so that they can pass it on to their patients.

How Can We Encourage People to Achieve Healthy Eating Patterns?

Research and knowledge about healthy nutrition abounds. Yet, despite individuals knowing what food is healthy, they continue to have unhealthy eating patterns. The question is not necessarily what is the healthiest way to eat, but how can we use the latest research in psychology to help people find a pathway toward eating well?

Promoting and Coaching Healthy Eating with the PERMA Elements

The focus of research on healthy eating has generally been on physical health outcomes. However, recently, researchers have been encouraged to extend this focus toward psychosocial benefits. Farmer and Cotter (2021) reviewed the literature relating to cooking and wellbeing and pointed to existing evidence on how they can contribute to wellbeing as defined by the PERMA model.

Participating in a five-session cooking class was associated with a boost of enjoyment during meal preparation (Adam et al., 2015). Equally, guiding participants through a series of three cooking classes showed an improvement in psychological wellbeing (Jyväkorpi et al., 2014). However, it is not necessarily the cooking course, but perhaps ways in which it is delivered that matters. In an Irish study with adults introduced to a cooking course, participants reported declines in wellbeing and increases in feeling inadequate as well as fear of introducing new menus to their families (Lavelle et al., 2016). Thus, the approach taken to introduce healthy food matters greatly.

One study presenting data from interviews conducted in the UK and the US explored the social and emotional dimensions of home cooking (Mills et al., 2020). Participants in this study reported that they associated "home cooking" with love, care, and nostalgia. "Cooking from scratch" was also an important part of home cooking, although they felt convenience foods could be included. Preparing raw ingredients could involve activities such as chopping. Although the authors did not explicitly make the connection, preparing foods from scratch could lead to the experience of psychological flow. Flow can occur when the challenge of cooking is increased and simultaneously matches their skill level (Csikszentmihalyi, 2021) and is a foundation for the engagement components of the PERMA model. However, there is limited research that directly explores cooking and engagement.

Cooking is often considered an opportunity for social connection, a time given to families and friends to share a moment together (Epley & Schroeder, 2014). Research with older women showed that they considered preparing a meal as a "gift" to their family (Sidenvall et al., 2000), as such cooking was an act of kindness. It is also an opportunity for parents to model healthy eating behavior to their children and promote healthy eating habits for their families (Berge et al., 2014). Therefore, the benefits of eating well go beyond nutrition.

The mindset used when preparing food and eating matters. Also, food could contribute to wellbeing via the meaning it provides for the family.

Creating the right environment for cooking is of utmost importance. When cooking is rushed, it may have a negative impact on wellbeing. On the other hand, when individuals have the time to prepare it and cook in the company of others, especially when the food they make is for others, the process of cooking becomes more meaningful (Daniels et al., 2012). That meaningfulness is amplified when parents are able to see what ingredients are in the meals they cook from scratch (Simmons & Chapman, 2012). This allows them to have control over their children's health. At the same time, for young people, cooking is an opportunity for developing independence. Thus, the process can become a growth-enhancing activity.

In relation to the achievement component of wellbeing, consistently, individuals prefer self-prepared food to food prepared by others (Dohle et al., 2014). This may be due to the sense of accomplishment they experience when making something. This is particularly important for young people. An ability to prepare their own meal is associated not only with increases in independence (Simmons & Champman, 2012), confidence, and wellbeing, but also decreases in depression (Utter et al., 2016). However, more research is required to identify the direct link between cooking and PERMA.

Applications of Positive Psychology with Healthy Eating for Positive Health

Several practices based on positive psychology frameworks and techniques can serve as essential tools for facilitating healthy eating, while at the same time promoting emotional and mental health. Integrating these applications in lifestyle medicine practice helps patients make progress toward positive health.

PERMA and Healthy Eating

Effectively coaching healthy eating represents a foundational aspect of lifestyle medicine and can be intentionally enhanced by applying the PERMA framework – positive emotions, engagement, relationships, meaning, and accomplishment. The list below shows examples of questions that emphasize each element of this well-known positive psychology framework.

Application of PERMA to Coach Healthy Eating

P—Positive emotions: Savor positive feelings that arise when you are enjoying your favorite healthy foods.
- What are positive memories of eating healthy foods when you were a child? Did you have a favorite fruit, for example, and what details do you recall about the experience of enjoying it?

- What kinds of healthy foods (e.g. vegetables, fruits, nuts), bring you the greatest joy and feeling of wellbeing and vitality?
- What are your happiest moments associated with eating? Where? With Whom? Recall those memories and look for ways to associate them with your current healthy eating plan.

E—Engagement (Flow): Notice how you can enhance the joy of eating your favorite healthy foods by mindfully eating them. Mindful eating involves becoming fully immersed in the experience, eating slowly, and being attentive to the flavors, aromas, textures, and sounds.
- Which of your senses can put you into a greater sense of flow when eating healthy food?
- How can you experience flow while preparing your favorite healthy meals?

R—Relationships: Identify how you can prepare and share your favorite healthy meals with others and increase your social interactions.
- What are traditional family meals or meals with friends that you can adjust to be both tasty and healthy?
- What people can you invite to cook and enjoy a healthy meal with you?

M—Meaning: Pay attention to how healthy eating aligns with your values and what is meaningful to you.
- What are meaningful ways you can engage your family and friends to enjoy and share healthy meals? How can that experience feel meaningful? For example, you may feel it is important to serve as a role model and help them become healthier and happier and live longer.
- How can eating healthy foods feel meaningful to you? For example, remember that eating healthy boosts your vitality so you can achieve your goals.

A—Achievement: Reflect on how progress toward a consistent healthy eating habit gives you a sense of accomplishment.
- What healthy recipes give you a genuine sense of accomplishment when you make them?
- What steps have you been making to shift toward eating healthy meals that give you a sense of pride and accomplishment?

Appreciative Inquiry for Healthy Eating

Appreciative inquiry is another positive psychology approach that can be used in health behavior change action planning to integrate healthy eating with positive emotions.

Discovery: What is good about healthy eating now?
- What kinds of healthy eating habits do you have now?
- What are some healthy recipes you make now?
- What are healthy restaurants or healthy items in restaurants that you enjoy?
- What strengths do you have that can help you achieve and maintain healthy eating habits?

Dream: What healthy eating changes are possible to create joy in your life?
- What new and different joyful eating habits are possible?
- What are additional ways to create joy while eating healthy food?

Design: What specific positive changes could you make in your eating habits?
- How could you eat more healthy foods that bring you joy?
- What strengths could you use to achieve this type of goal?
- With whom could you prepare and share healthy food, i.e. feed your body and soul by connecting with others over healthy meals?

Destiny: What positive changes are you confident you can make in your eating habits now?
- What action plan for eating healthy will give you a sense of joy, pride, or other positive feelings?
- Which strengths will you use to achieve your action plan?
- What are healthy ways you can reward yourself for achieving your action plan?

Integrating Positive Health into Lifestyle Medicine Competencies: Nutrition Science, Assessment, and Prescription

As health practitioners increase their knowledge and skills for clinical practice that emphasizes lifestyle medicine, the lifestyle medicine competencies (Lianov et al., 2022) offer a guide for honing and refining those skills. Several of the competencies in the Nutrition Science, Assessment, and Prescription section do not explicitly cite the connection between nutrition and emotional and mental health. You can advance your skills by making sure to include this connection. The list below highlights several competencies in this section with adjustments to help you practice "lifestyle medicine from the inside out."

- When assessing food intake patterns and nutrients of deficit and excess, ask which foods bring forth positive emotions. Any healthy food that increases positive emotions may offer a starting point for making successful changes.

- In a summary of the health impact of prominent dietary patterns, including plant-predominant and non–plant-predominant patterns, highlight the impact of these patterns on mental and emotional wellbeing, as well as physical wellbeing.
- When describing the practice of culinary medicine and its role in sustainable healthy eating behavior, including how positive psychology principles can be integrated, such as the experience of flow when chopping vegetables and preparing meals with others to increase positivity resonance.
- In a summary of the major studies of nutrition in the prevention, treatment, and reversal of hyperlipidemia, cardiovascular disease, prediabetes, diabetes, hypertension, obesity, and cancer, add studies of the nutritional impact on positive emotions, depression, mental disorders, and emotional wellbeing.
- Develop nutrition prescriptions based on science that shows how nutrition can address the pathophysiology of most chronic diseases, as well as many mental and emotional conditions, including inflammation, oxidation, glycosylation, epigenetic expression, and the microbiome.
- When writing evidence-based nutrition prescriptions, discuss with patients how these prescriptions treat mental health conditions and increase positive emotions, which reinforce the upward spiral of lifestyle change, or include written reminders about steps to increase positive emotions during healthy eating.

Table 3.2 lists the lifestyle medicine competencies in nutrition science, assessment, and prescription in the left column. It suggests the additions in the right column to expand the competency for positive health practice.

Perspectives on Practicing Lifestyle Medicine from the Inside Out – Healthy Eating

Our own experiences and biases impact our success in helping patients make desired changes. The link between diet and health goes well beyond the ingredients in the food. Social, cultural, economic, and identity aspects of food influence the ultimate success of the change in eating patterns, as well as its outcomes (Lee et al., 2023). In an innovative qualitative study, researchers uncovered three themes for the food and mood relationship.

1 Social context: familial and cultural influences of food and mood
2 Social economics: time, finance, and food security
3 Food nostalgia: memories about food that impact mood

Practicing lifestyle medicine from the inside out can involve addressing these themes using positive psychology principles. This approach carries the

Table 3.2 Positive health in lifestyle medicine competencies: nutrition science, assessment, and prescription

Lifestyle medicine competency	Positive health expansion
Assess food intake patterns and nutrients of deficit and excess	Assess patterns of eating that increase positive emotions
Summarize the health impact of prominent dietary patterns, including plant-predominant and non–plant-predominant patterns	Summarize the impact of healthy eating patterns on mental and emotional wellbeing, as well as physical wellbeing
Describe the practice of culinary medicine and its role in sustainable healthy eating behavior	Describe how positive psychology principles can be integrated into culinary medicine, e.g. the experience of flow when chopping vegetables and positivity resonance when preparing meals with others
Summarize the major studies of nutrition in the prevention, treatment, and reversal of hyperlipidemia, cardiovascular disease, prediabetes, diabetes, hypertension, obesity, and cancer	Summarize studies of the impact of nutrition on positive emotions, depression, mental disorders, and emotional wellbeing
Apply nutrition prescriptions based on science that shows how nutrition can address the pathophysiology of most chronic diseases, including inflammation, oxidation, glycosylation, epigenetic expression, and the microbiome	Apply nutrition prescriptions based on science to address mental and emotional conditions and increase positive emotions
Demonstrate the ability to write evidence-based nutrition prescriptions	Demonstrate the ability to write prescriptions that treat mental health conditions and increase positive emotions, which reinforce the upward spiral of lifestyle change; demonstrate the ability to write the steps for increasing positive emotions during healthy eating

potential to help patients move forward from patterns that keep them stuck in old eating behaviors. Although the positive psychology approach may not directly address barriers such as social economics, by leveraging other powerful supports, such as social context, and increasing positive emotions, the individual may increase their capacity to problem-solve these barriers.

Many of us can relate to experiences during celebratory occasions with positive emotions when we might eat unhealthy food and overeat. Yet, the literature emphasizes the role of positive emotions in healthy eating. In addition to improved problem-solving, other mechanisms link positive psychology with healthy eating. A recent qualitative study of individuals with metabolic syndrome echoes the connection between positive psychology and healthy eating via several themes. Eating healthfully can prevent negative emotions, positive psychology constructs can increase healthy eating behaviors, and positive emotions can lead to an upward spiral of healthy eating behavior change (Carrillo et al., 2022).

As you recommend to a patient a change in eating habits, first, self-reflect honestly. What experiences have you had with making a transition to healthy eating? What kind of self-talk and support were most effective to help you make the change? How do you feel about the specific healthy eating prescription you are making? Highlight and savor positive emotions that you notice when envisioning eating this way. What strengths did you use to make a meaningful change?

This kind of honest self-reflection will help you connect with the patient from a place of understanding. Share those experiences with the patient, when feasible, as you introduce the prescription and facilitate the healthy eating change. The positivity resonance that may result can help the patient bring forth positive emotions later when following this eating pattern.

Practice Tools for Applying Positive Psychology to Healthy Eating

You can prescribe a healthy eating goal supported with positive psychology according to TAF – type of food, amount of food, and frequency of consuming that food. The TAF prescription can be enhanced with positive psychology approaches – by adding the three S's – sharing, strengths, and savoring. The first S is for sharing: With whom can you share this goal? The second S is for strengths: What strengths can you use to help you achieve this goal? The third S is for savoring: Pay attention to positive feelings (and flavors!) while accomplishing this goal. This kind of prescription bridges the basic nutrition prescription with positive psychology supports that can powerfully change the dialogue about making behavior changes. A health coach (or health team member in the coaching role) can help the patient create an action plan based on what the patient is ready to do as a first step toward meeting the prescription goal. Emphasizing the three Ss in the action plan, not only spells out feasible first steps but also concretely brings attention to factors that can support progress.

Example: Positive Psychology-Based Broccoli Prescription

Broccoli [type]
One serving/about the size of a fist [amount]
3x weekly [frequency]

Meet this goal with your support:

- Sharing: Identify someone with whom can you share this goal
- Strengths: Use your strengths to help you achieve this goal
- Savoring: Pay attention to positive feelings (and flavors!) while accomplishing this goal

REFILLS: Unlimited

The provider or one of the health team members can help the patient identify an action plan they are ready for and confident at a level of 7 or above on a scale of 1 (least confident) to 10 (most confident) they can achieve. They can include how they will use sharing, strengths, and savoring to support the plan.

Action Plan Example: I will include in my evening meal one serving of broccoli every other day. I will ask my partner to help remind me about this goal when we go grocery shopping and see if she is willing to add broccoli to her meals. I'll use my strengths of kindness to help me with this goal. I think if I role model healthy eating, I can help her health too. I look forward to savoring the positive feelings of pride when I achieve this goal and help my partner.

Specific PPIs to Promote Healthy Eating Behaviors

Several additional PPIs have been used to promote healthy eating behaviors, including gratitude, self-compassion, and mindfulness.

Gratitude

Gratitude practice focuses on the positive aspects of life, including the things for which we are thankful. It can be effective in promoting healthy eating behaviors by helping individuals to appreciate the positive aspects of healthy eating, such as the enjoyment of delicious and nutritious food. For example, in one study of adolescents and young adults, those assigned to the gratitude practice reported healthy eating behavior over time, compared to the control group assigned to list daily activities (Fritz et al., 2019)

Self-Compassion

Self-compassion, the practice of treating oneself with kindness and understanding, especially during difficult times, represents an essential practice during any behavior change. It has been found to be effective in promoting healthy eating behaviors by reducing self-criticism and negative emotions related to food and eating. One study reported that participants who were instructed to practice self-compassion to alleviate stress reported healthier eating habits (Yanjuan et al., 2020). Healthy eating when practicing self-compassion may also be related to greater self-acceptance and less negative emotions about their relationship to food.

Mindfulness

Mindfulness, the practice of being present at the moment and paying attention to one's thoughts and feelings without judgment, has been found to be effective in promoting healthy eating behaviors. Mindfulness during eating can help individuals become more aware of their hunger and fullness cues, as well as their emotional triggers for eating. Study participants who were instructed to practice mindfulness when eating reported greater satisfaction with their meals and greater awareness of their hunger and fullness cues (Mantzios & Wilson, 2015).

Other PPIs that have been used to promote healthy eating behaviors include positive self-talk (Rose et al., 2022), goal-setting both for specific eating habits and other healthy habit and life goals (Turner-McGrievy et al., 2014), and social support (Yoshikawa et al., 2021). These interventions can help individuals develop positive healthy eating habits and routines and build the motivation and support needed to sustain these habits.

Case Study of Positive Health Approaches for Healthy Eating

This case study focuses on how positive psychology approaches can support the healthy eating pillar. Chapters 4–8 include case studies on addressing the other healthy lifestyle pillars. Chapter 11 offers a case study comparing positive health with lifestyle medicine and traditional healthcare approaches.

Patient Background: Joe is a 52-year-old white, single man who has been diagnosed with hypercholesterolemia and hypertension. He is overweight with a body mass index of 25 and reports feeling lethargic and stressed about a "difficult" customer. His main activity outside of his accounting job is watching sports. He split up with his partner two years ago and occasionally dates, but mostly keeps to himself. Both of his parents passed away five years earlier and he has no siblings. He is

currently taking medications to control his blood pressure and cholesterol without significant improvement.

Assessment: The provider assesses Joe's dietary habits along with
other health habits. She holds an authentic conversation with Joe about
what he wants to accomplish regarding his health and wellbeing. Joe
shares that he'd like to start feeling less stressed and more energetic
overall so that he'd feel up for going to a ballgame with a buddy he's
not seen in a q long time.

Treatment Plan: The provider recommends a comprehensive
healthy lifestyle plan. She recommends a predominantly whole food
plant-based diet, along with the other pillars of a healthy lifestyle, to
improve his blood pressure and cholesterol, as well as enhance his
emotional wellbeing. She refers Joe to the dietician on the health team.

Intervention from the Inside Out: The dietitian conducts an in-depth
assessment of Joe's dietary habits and identifies that he consumes a
high-fat, high-cholesterol diet with minimal intake of fruits and vegetables. She also suggests strategies for increasing the intake of these
foods and then applies health coaching techniques that leverage positive psychology. The following steps are implemented:

1 Nutrition education: The dietitian explains the benefits of a whole
   food plant-based diet, such as reducing inflammation and improving his blood pressure and cholesterol, heart health, as well as his
   mental and emotional health.
2 Meal planning: The prescription recommends shifting the eating
   pattern to at least three-fourths of his caloric intake coming from
   plant-based whole foods. The dietitian develops a meal plan of a variety of plant-based foods, such as fruits, vegetables, whole grains,
   legumes, nuts, and seeds. The plan includes recipes and cooking
   tips and is divided into steps for reaching the overall goal. The first
   recommended step is adding at least two servings of vegetables to
   each lunch and dinner meal.
3 Behavioral change strategies with positive psychology: The dietitian checks Joe's readiness and confidence to shift his eating pattern, starting with his confidence to add at least two servings of
   vegetables to each lunch and dinner meal. Joe's confidence level
   is 8 on a scale of 1 to 10 that he could add one serving to each
   lunch and dinner four days a week. He recalls that he used to enjoy
   broccoli with hot sauce in his youth and decides to try that again.

They also discuss positive psychological supports for achieving this plan.

- Sharing: With whom can you share this goal? *My nephew who is studying to become a nurse at a college in another state; occasionally chat about recent sports games.*
- Strengths: What strengths can you use to help you achieve this goal? *Perseverance to get back on track if I find I am not being consistent with the plan.*
- Savoring: What positive feelings (and flavors!) do you anticipate? *Feeling proud about taking care of myself.*
- Success celebration: How can you celebrate partial successes as you achieve your goal? *Attend a ballgame.*

4 PPIs: The dietitian encourages Joe to practice mindfulness and notice positive experiences while eating. This process involves being present and attentive while eating, savoring the flavors and textures of the food, and expressing gratitude for the nourishment it provides. Joe can increase his natural, unforced motivation to eat healthy by paying attention to positive experiences and feelings while doing so.

Outcome: After three months of adding vegetables to his meals, Joe's blood pressure and cholesterol levels decreased, and he lost five pounds. He also reports feeling more energetic. The dietitian conducts a follow-up assessment and notes that he is eating a serving of vegetables with most meals and has developed a greater appreciation for plant-based foods. They discuss the next steps, such as increasing the servings of vegetables and decreasing his meat consumption. Joe shares that he has a ballgame coming up that he will be attending with his buddy.

Key Take-Aways: This case demonstrates the important link between healthy lifestyles and positive emotions for improving physical and mental health outcomes. Incorporating positive psychology approaches – the three Ss of sharing, strengths, and savoring – into behavioral change strategies, along with PPIs, such as mindfulness and gratitude practices, can enhance positive emotions and physical health outcomes, which reinforce each other. The health team's collaborative approach to helping Joe emphasize the positive aspects of making change and leveraging positive emotions was crucial in achieving his healthy eating goal.

Conclusion

Positive emotions and healthy eating have a reciprocal and reinforcing relationship. Practicing lifestyle medicine from the inside out emphasizes positive psychology principles and serves as a valuable approach to promoting healthy eating behaviors. By leveraging the patient's positive experiences and supports, focusing on the positive aspects of healthy eating, identifying strengths and values related to healthy eating, and using PPIs such as gratitude, self-compassion, and mindfulness, to increase positive emotions that boost problem-solving, individuals can develop healthy eating habits and routines. As healthy eating habits are built and maintained, positive emotions can be increased in an upward spiral of healthy eating changes. Although this practice approach shows much promise, further research is needed to explore the effectiveness of the applications of these principles and interventions in healthcare settings for different medical conditions and patient populations.

References

Adam, M., Young-Wolff, K. C., & Konar, E., & Winkleby, M. (2015). Massive open online nutrition and cooking course for improved eating behaviors and meal composition. *Int J Behav Nutr Phys Act, 12*, 143. https://doi.org/10.1186/s12966-015-0305-2

Ait-Hadad, W., Bénard, M., & Shankland, R., Kesse-Guyot, E., Robert, T., Touvier, M., Hercberg, S., Buscail, C., & Péneau S. (2020). Optimism is associated with diet quality, food group consumption and snacking behavior in a general population. *Nutr J., 19*(1), 6. https://doi.org/10.1186/s12937-020-0522-7

Berge, J. M., Rowley, S., Trofholz, A., Hanson, C., Rueter, M., MacLehose, R. F., & Neumark-Sztainer, D. (2014). Childhood obesity and interpersonal dynamics during family meals. *Pediatrics, 134*(5), 923–932. https://doi.org/10.1542/peds.2014-1936.

Blanchflower, D. G., Oswald, A. J., & Stewart-Brown, S. (2013). Is psychological well-being linked to the consumption of fruit and vegetables? *Social Indicators Research, 114*(3), 785–801. https://doi.org/10.1007/s11205-012-0173-y.

Block, L. G., Grier, S. A., Childers, T. L., Davis, B., Ebert, J. E. J., Kumanyika, S., Laczniak, R. N., Machin, J. E., Motley, C. M., Peracchio, L., Pettigrew, S., Scott, M., & van Ginkel Bieshaar, M. N. G. (2011). From nutrients to nurturance: A conceptual introduction to food well-being. *Journal of Public Policy & Marketing, 30*(1), 5–13. https://doi.org/10.1509/jppm.30.1.5.

Conner, T. S. & Silvia, P. J. (2015). Creative days: A daily diary study of emotion, personality, and everyday creativity. Psychology of Aesthetics, Creativity, and the Arts, 9(4), 463–470. https://doi.org/10.1080/10400419.2022.2122371

Csikszentmihalyi, M. (2021). Flow: A component of the good life. In A. Kostić, & D. Chadee (Eds.), *Positive psychology: An international perspective* (pp. 193–200). Wiley Blackwell.

Daniels, S., Glorieux, I., Minnen, J., & van Tienoven, T. P. (2012). More than preparing a meal? Concerning the meanings of home cooking. *Appetite, 58*(3), 1050–1056. https://doi.org/10.1016/j.appet.2012.02.040.

Dohle, S., Rall, S., & Siegrist, M. (2014). I cooked it myself: Preparing food increases liking and consumption. *Food Quality and Preference, 33*, 14–16. https://doi.org/ 10.1016/j.foodqual.2013.11.001

Drake, A., Doré, B., & Falk, E. B., Zurn, P., Bassett, D. S., & Lydon-Staley, D. M. (2022). Daily stressor-related negative mood and its associations with flourishing and daily curiosity. *J Happiness Stud., 23*, 423–438. https://doi.org/10.1007/ s10902-021-00404-2

Fararouei, M., Brown, I. J., Akbartabar, T. M., Estakhrian, H. R., & Jafari, J. (2013). Happiness and health behavior in Iranian adolescent girls. *J Adolesc., 36*(6), 1187–1192. https://doi.org/10.3389/fpsyg.2021.560578

Farmer, N., & Cotter, E. W. (2021). Well-being and cooking behavior: Using the positive emotion, engagement, relationships, meaning, and accomplishment (PERMA) model as a theoretical framework. *Frontiers in Psychology, 12*, 560578.

Frates, B., Bonnet, J. P., Joseph, R., & Peterson, J. A. (2020*). Lifestyle medicine handbook, an introduction to the power of healthy habits.* Healthy Learning.

Fritz, M. M., Armento, C. N., Walsh, L. C., & Lyubomirsky, S. (2019). Gratitude facilitates healthy behavior in adolescents and young adults. *Journal of Experimental Social Psychology, 81*, 4–14. https://doi.org/10.1016/j.jesp.2018.08.011

Gardner, M. P., Wansink, B., Kim, J., & Park, S.-B. (2014). Better moods for better eating? How mood influences food choice. *Journal of Consumer Psychology, 24*(3), 320–335. https://doi.org/10.1016/j.jcps.2014.01.001.

Hingle, M. D., Wertheim, B. C., & Tindle, H. A. (2014). Optimism and diet quality in the Women's health initiative. *J Acad Nutr Diet, 114*(7), 1036–1045. https://doi.org/ 10.1016/j.jand.2013.12.018.

Ho, H. C. Y., Mui, M. W., Wan, A., Yew, C. W., & Lam, T. H. (2020). Happy family kitchen movement A cluster randomized controlled trail of a community-based family holistic intervention in Hong Kong. Journal of Happiness Studies, *21*, 15–36. https://doi.org/10.1007/s10902-018-00071-w

Jyväkorpi, S., Pitkälä, K., Kautiainen, H., Puranen, T., Laakkonen, M., & Suominen, M. (2014). Nutrition education and cooking classes improve diet quality, nutrient intake, and psychological well-being of home-dwelling older people—A pilot study. *Morb. Mortal, 1*, 4–8.

Kashdan, T. B. (2009). *Curious: Discover the missing ingredient to a fulfilling life.* Harper Collins Publishers.

Lavelle, F., Spence, M., & Hollywood, L., McGowan, L., Surgenor, D., McCloat, A., Mooney, E., Caraher, M., Raats, M., & Dean, M. (2016). Learning cooking skills at different ages: A cross-sectional study. *Int J Behav Nutr Phys Act 13, 119*. https://doi. org/10.1186/s12966-016-0446-y

Lee, M. F., Angus, D., Walsh, H., & Sargeant, S. (2023). "Maybe it's not just the food?" A food and mood focus group study. *Int J Environ Res Public Health, 20*(3), 2011. https://doi.org/10.3390/ijerph20032011.

Lesani, A., Mohammadpoorasl, A., Javadi, M., Esfeh, J. M., & Fakhari, A. (2016). Eating breakfast, fruit and vegetable intake and their relation with happiness in college students. *Eating and Weight Disorders, 21*(4), 645–651. https://doi.org/10.1007/ s40519-016-0261-0.

Li, Y., Deng, J., Lou, X., Wang, H., & Wang, Y. (2019) A daily diary of the relationships among daily self-compassion, perceived stress and healthpromoting behaviors. *Int J Psychol., 55*(3), 364–372. https://doi.org/10.1002/ijop.12610

Lianov, L. S., Adamson, K., Kelly, J. H., Mathews, S., Palma, M., & Rea, B. L. (2022). Lifestyle medicine core competencies: 2022 update. *Am J Lifestyle Med, 16*(6), 734–739. https://doi.org/10.1177/15598276221121580

Macht, M., Meininger, J., & Roth, J. (2005). The pleasures of eating: A qualitative analysis. *J Happiness Stud, 6,* 137–160. https://doi.org/10.1007/s10902-005-0287-x

Magallares, A., & Pais-Ribeiro, J. L. (2014). Mental health and obesity: A meta-analysis. *Applied Research in Quality of Life, 9*(2), 295–308. https://doi.org/10.1007/s11482-013-9226-x.

Messer, M., Anderon, C., & Linardon, J. (2021). Self-compassion explains substantially more variance in eating disorder psychopathology and associated impairment than mindfulness. *Body Image,* 36, 27–33. https://doi.org/10.1016/j.bodyim.2020.10.002

Mills, S. D. H., Wolfson, J. A., Wrieden, W. L., Brown, H., White, M., & Adams, J. (2020). Perceptions of "home-cooking": A qualitative analysis from the United Kingdom and the United States. *Nutrients, 12*(1), 198. https://doi.org/10.3390/nu12010198.

Mantzios, M., & Wilson, J. C. (2015). Mindfulness, eating behaviors, and obesity: A review and reflection on current findings. *Curr Obes Rep, 4*(1), 141–146. https://doi.org/10.1007/s13679-014-0131-x.

Mujcic, R., & Oswald, A. J. (2016). Evolution of well-being and happiness after increases in consumption of fruit and vegetables. *Am J Public Health, 106*(8), 1504–1510. https://doi.org/10.2105/AJPH.2016.303260.

Neff, K. D. (2003). Self-compassion: An alternative conceptualization of a healthy attitude toward oneself. *Self and Identity, 2*(2), 85–101. https://doi.org/10.1080/15298860309032.

Neff, K. D. (2023). Self Compassion guided practices and exercises. Retrieved from: https://self-compassion.org/category/exercises/#:~:text=Keeping%20a%20daily%20journal%20in,part%20of%20your%20daily%20life.

Neff, K. D., Knox, M. C., Long, P., & Gregory, K. (2020). Caring for others without losing yourself: An adaptation of the mindful self-compassion program for healthcare communities. *J. Clin. Psychol., 76,* 1543–1562. https://doi.org/10.1002/jclp.23007

Pänkäläinen, M., Fogelholm, M., Valve, R., Kamoman, O., Kauppi, M., Lappalainen, E., & Hintikka, J. (2018). Pessimism, diet, and the ability to improve dietary habits: A three-year follow-up study among middle-aged and older Finnish men and women. *Nutr J, 17*(1), 92. https://doi.org/10.1186/s12937-018-0400-8.

Phelan, S. M., Burgess, D. J., Yeazel, M. W., Hellerstedt, W. L., Griffin, J. M., & van Ryn, M. (2015). Impact of weight bias and stigma on quality of care and outcomes for patients with obesity. *Obesity Reviews: An Official Journal of the International Association for the Study of Obesity, 16*(4), 319–326. https://doi.org/10.1111/obr.12266.

Phillips, W. J. & Hine, D. W. (2019). Self-compassion, physical health, and health behavior: a meta-analysis. Health Psychology Reviews. 15(1), 113–139. https://doi.org/10.1080/17437199.2019.1705872

Prendergast, K. B., Mackay, L. M., & Schofield, G. M. (2016). The clustering of lifestyle behaviours in New Zealand and their relationship with optimal wellbeing. *Int. J. Behav. Med., 23,* 571–579. https://doi.org/10.1007/s12529-016-9552-0

Puhl, R. M., & Latner, J. D. (2007). Stigma, obesity, and the health of the nation's children. *Psychological Bulletin, 133*(4), 557–580. https://doi.org/10.1037/0033-2909.133.4.557.

Rose, J., Pedrazzi, R., & Dombroski, S. U. (2022). Examining dietary self-talk content and context for discretionary snacking behavior: A qualitative interview study. *Health Psychol Behav Med, 10*(1), 399–414. https://doi.org/10.1080/21642850.202 2.2053686.

Simmons, D., & Chapman, G. E. (2012). The significance of home cooking within families. *British Food Journal, 114*(8), 1184–1195. https://doi.org/10.1108/0007070 1211252110.

Sarin, S., Motta, M., & Gobble, J. E. (2022). *The practitioner's guide to lifestyle medicine*. Healthy Learning.

Sidenvall, B., Nydahl, M., & Fjellström, C. (2000). The meal as a gift—The meaning of cooking among retired women. *Journal of Applied Gerontology, 19*(4), 405–423. https://doi.org/10.1177/073346480001900403.

Stranges, S., Samaraweera, P. C., & Taggart, F., et al. (2014). Major health-related behaviours and mental well-being in The general population: The health survey for England. *BMJ Open, 4*, e005878. https://doi.org/10.1136/bmjopen-2014-005878

Turner-McGrievy, G. M., Wright, J. A., & Migneault, J. P., et al. (2014). The interaction between dietary and life goals: Using goal systems theory to explore healthy diet and life goals. *Health Psychol Behav Med., 2*(1), 759–769. https://doi.org/10.1080/2164 2850.2014.927737

Utter, J., Denny, S., Lucassen, M., & Dyson, B. (2016). Adolescent cooking abilities and behaviors: Associations with nutrition and emotional well-being. *Journal of Nutrition Education and Behavior, 48*(1), 35–41. https://doi.org/10.1016/j.jneb.2015.08.016.

Van Cappellen, P., Rice, E. L., & Catalino, L. I., et al. (2018) Positive affective processes underlie positive health behavior change. *Psychol Health., 33*(1), 77–97. https://doi.org/10.1080/08870446.2017.1320798

Warner, R., Frye, K., Morrell, J., & Carey, G. (2017). Fruit and vegetable intake predicts positive affect. *Journal of Happiness Studies, 18*(3), 809–826. https://doi.org/10.1007/s10902-016-9749-6.

Whatnall, M. C., Patterson, A. J., Siew, Y. Y., Kay-Lambkin, F., & Hutchesson, M. J. (2019). Are psychological distress and resilience associated with dietary intake among Australian university students? *Int J Environ Res Public Health, 16*(21), 4099. https://doi.org/10.3390/ijerph16214099.

White, B. A., Horwath, C. C., & Conner, T. S. (2013). Many apples a day keep the blues away–daily experiences of negative and positive affect and food consumption in young adults. *British Journal of Health Psychology, 18*(4), 782–798. https://doi.org/10.1111/bjhp.12021.

Yoshikawa, A., Smith, M.L., Lee, S., Towne., S. D., & Ory, M.G. (2021). The role of improved social support for healthy eating in a lifestyle intervention: Telexercise select. *Public Health Nutr., 24*(1), 146–156. https://doi.org/10.1017/S1368980020002700

4 Positive Psychology and Physical Activity for Positive Health

Chapter Overview

This chapter reviews the relationship between physical activity, positive emotions, and positive psychology interventions with highlights from scientific literature. Clinical coaching applications of the PERMA model and other practical clinical techniques are presented for leveraging positive psychology to promote physical activity and positive health. In turn, the power of physical activity to drive positive emotions and wellbeing is highlighted.

Introduction

Positive psychology interventions can help individuals increase positive emotions and develop their character strengths, such as perseverance, self-control, and gratitude. These activities boost resilience and improve behaviors, including physical activity, leading to better health outcomes. The combination of positive psychology interventions and physical activity can have a synergistic and powerful effect on wellbeing.

Physical Activity Improves Physical and Mental Health and Increases Positive Affect

Physical activity, such as walking, running, swimming, weightlifting, and yoga – has been linked to numerous health benefits – including reducing the risk of chronic diseases, improving mental and emotional health, and promoting longevity (Piercy et al., 2018). Empirical studies strongly support these health benefits for populations with and without mental illness. For example, physical activity has been shown to be effective both in reducing risk for and treating depression extensive scientific literature (Babyak et al., 2000; Blake, 2012;

DOI: 10.4324/9781003428909-4

Blumenthal et al., 2007; Carek et al., 2011; Cooney et al., 2013; Dinas et al., 2011; Ernst et al., 2006; Hallgren et al., 2017; Mammen & Faulkner, 2013; McKercher et al., 2014; Rimer et al., 2012). In fact, outcomes resulting from the treatment of depression with physical activity have been shown to be comparable to those of cognitive therapy (Rimer et al., 2012). In some cases, physical activity is slightly more effective when compared with standard treatments, including medication (Cooney et al., 2013).

Physical activity confers positive effects on mental health and subjective wellbeing through biochemical pathways – increases in endorphins, reduction in cortisol levels, oxidative stress and inflammation, and alteration in neurotransmitter function – as well as cognitive and emotional mechanisms, such as boosts in self-esteem, self-efficacy, and social support and including positive psychology constructs, such as a sense of purpose (Blake, 2012; Kandola et al., 2019). Interestingly, another mechanism by which positive psychology constructs play a role in mental health to consider is a link between loneliness and physical activity. Loneliness is a risk factor for reduced physical activity among older adults, and this risk can, in part, be countered with interventions that increase positive emotions (McCauley et al, 2003, Newall et al., 2012). Moreover, positive emotions can also increase psychosocial resources known to improve mental wellbeing and support and enhance other elements of wellbeing (Hogan et al., 2015).

Improvements in mood in healthy adults can be seen with as little as 10 minutes of exercise (Hansen et al., 2001), and more recently the recommendations support fitting any activity into one's day, such as parking farther away or taking stairs (Piercy et al., 2018). Physical movement, which can be prompted through smartphones and internet-interventions, in daily routines can contribute to better moods (Lathia et al., 2017, Hartman et al, 2017). Looking beyond mental illness treatment and improving moods, research has also found an association between the role of physical activity in promoting positive emotions (Li et al., 2022) and character strengths (Proyer et al., 2013) for enhancing wellbeing and achieving positive health.

Positive Emotions and Positive Psychology Interventions Can Promote Physical Activity

Despite the benefits of physical activity, many individuals struggle with achieving recommended levels of physical activity due to barriers such as lack of time, motivation, concerns about environmental air pollution and personal safety, and lack of resources (Koh et al., 2022). Interventions for increasing physical activity levels and addressing these barriers can be made more effective through positive psychology approaches.

Research has shown that the experience of positive emotions during physical activity and exercise can increase future physical activity (Rhodes & Kates, 2015). Other researchers have found that interventions to increase positive emotions and address factors that lead to negative affect have the potential to serve as effective supports to help individuals achieve physical activity goals (Feig et al., 2022). When individuals experience positive emotions during physical activity, the upward spiral of lifestyle change leads to reinforcing this health behavior change. Positive emotions can enhance the experience of physical activity, making it more enjoyable and increasing motivation to do this activity again. Moreover, an 11-year prospective study reported an association between increased psychological wellbeing and subsequent higher levels of physical activity. (Kim et al., 2017a).

Optimism and Physical Activity

Optimistic thinking is associated with an increase in physical activity (Chen et al., 2023). In studies with young people and older patients, those who practice optimistic thinking are significantly more likely to be physically active (Cekin, 2015; Kim et al., 2017b). Optimists tend to persevere more than pessimists (Carver & Scheier, 2014), as such, they are more likely to stick with their physical regime than pessimists. The reason for it may lie in experiencing more positive emotions resulting from optimism. When experiencing negative emotions, it is hard to maintain the practice. Thus, optimism is a pathway for encouraging regular physical activity practice.

Positive Psychology Interventions and Physical Activity

Positive psychology interventions can be used as single activities or as part of a wellbeing program that runs over several weeks, often changing activities each week. Such a program was developed for patients with type 2 diabetes, for whom physical activity is crucial to achieving glycemic control and overall health (Huffman et al., 2021; Millstein et al., 2022). The program aimed to help patients find personally meaningful motivation to engage in physical activity. The researchers have applied an eight-week program comprising an activity for motivational interviewing and another from positive psychology each week. Positive psychology activities ranged from expressing gratitude for positive events during the week, writing a gratitude letter to someone and thanking them for their kindness, recalling past successes, and using personal strengths in daily life. Those who took part in the program increased their engagement in physical activity, that is, the number of steps for up to 24 weeks. Thus, a program like this can be beneficial for patients' health and wellbeing.

Enjoyable and Meaningful Activities (Adapted from Millstein et al., 2022)

This week make sure to engage in an enjoyable activity on your own, another enjoyable activity with someone, and an activity that has a deep meaning to you.

Applications of Positive Psychology in Physical Activity for Positive Health

Physical activity represents a foundational element of lifestyle medicine, which can be supported through the applications of a number of positive psychology strategies. A few of these are introduced here, along with a suggested expansion of lifestyle medicine to highlight positive health.

Coaching Physical Activity with PERMA

A practitioner can use the PERMA model to coach behavior change in physical activity. The list below shows examples of questions that emphasize each element of the model in the context of physical activity.

Application of PERMA for Increasing Physical Activity

P—Positive emotions: Savor positive feelings that arise when you are doing any form of movement and physical activity.
- What positive childhood memories do you have of being physically active?
- What type of physical activity brings you the greatest feeling of vitality?
- What setting for physical activity is associated with the greatest positive emotions? For example, being active outside in nature or in a gym or exercise class surrounded by others.

E—Engagement (Flow): Look for physical activities that make you fully attentive to what you are doing.
- Which physical activities bring you into a state of flow so that you lose track of time and your surroundings, focused on the present?
- How can you do a favorite physical activity so that you become fully attentive to the activity?

R—Relationships: Identify how physical activity can be done with others and how you can increase social interactions by engaging in physical activities together.
- What physical activities can you do with or around others? Examples: classes, neighborhood walking groups, and sports
- What physical activities can you do with people who are important to you? Examples: an evening walk with your partner, a ball game with your children, hiking with friends

M—Meaning: Pay attention to how being physically active aligns with your values and what feels meaningful.
- What physical activities could you do that add meaning to your life? Examples: volunteering at a local food bank where you move boxes of food or working in a community garden

- What physical activities can you do to align with your values? Example: riding your bike to work instead of driving a gas-powered car to help slow climate change or running in a race to raise money for your daughter's school

A—Achievement: Reflect on how progress toward the goal gives you a sense of accomplishment.
- What types of physical activities provide you with a genuine sense of accomplishment? Examples: climbing a mountain, bicycling a certain distance, competing in a race, running a marathon
- What physical activity action plan will allow you to track and celebrate each success along the way to your ultimate goal?

Appreciative Inquiry for Increasing Physical Activity

The positive psychology framework of appreciative inquiry can be tailored to facilitate physical activity action plans by integrating positive psychology principles into the process.

Discovery: What is good now? What physical activities do you do now that you can celebrate?
- What kinds of regular physical activity habits do you like to engage in now?
- What are your favorite forms of physical activity, whether you do them regularly or occasionally?
- Which types of physical movement do you do that give you a sense of vitality and joy?
- Which strengths do you use to help you maintain physical activity habits?

Dream: What physical activity changes that would create joy in life are possible?
- What new fun and invigorating physical activities sound interesting?
- What are possible ways to increase one's level of physical activity?

Design: What changes in your physical activity habits are feasible?
- How could you bring more joyful physical activity into your routine?
- What strengths could you use to achieve this goal?
- With whom could you engage in physical activities and build positive social connections?

Destiny: What positive changes are you confident you can make in your physical activity habits?
- What action plan for increasing physical activity will give you a sense of joy, pride, or other positive feelings?

- Which strengths will you use to achieve your action plan?
- What are healthy ways you can reward yourself for achieving your action plan?

Integrating Positive Health into Lifestyle Medicine Competencies: Physical Activity Science, Assessment, and Prescription

The lifestyle medicine competencies (Lianov et al., 2022) offer guidance for essential practice skills. You can advance your skills by making sure to include the connection between mental and emotional health, especially positive emotions, and physical activity. The list below highlights several competencies in this section with suggested adjustments to help you practice lifestyle medicine from the inside out to achieve positive health.

- When examining the evidence and pathophysiology between physical activity components and health outcomes, include the evidence for the impact of physical activity on mental and emotional health outcomes.
- When describing the benefits of physical activity in preventing or treating disease in special populations (such as healthy older adults, pregnant women, children and adolescents, persons with obesity or disability, cardiovascular disease, diabetes, cancer, disability, and stroke) include the benefits of mental and emotional health.
- When integrating key physical activity assessment tools into clinical practice, include assessment of positive experiences and positive emotions.
- When integrating evidence from relevant physical activity literature into treatment protocols for management, remission, or reversal in patients with diabetes, cancer, cardiovascular, and cerebrovascular disease, include the evidence from physical activity literature on treatment protocols for improving mental and emotional health outcomes, increasing resilience and achieving positive health.

Table 4.1 lists the lifestyle medicine competencies in the left column and suggests additional skills and knowledge to expand the pillar of physical activity for achieving positive health.

Perspectives on Practicing Lifestyle Medicine from the Inside Out – Physical Activity

As with other health behaviors, health providers' experiences and biases impact success in helping patients make desired changes. We can increase our success by drawing from personal struggles that were shifted through positive experiences and emotions that we associate with physical activity. Practicing lifestyle medicine from the inside out involves harnessing the positive psychology approach to help patients achieve and maintain their physical activity action plans. In fact, physical activity changes have a powerful link with positive emotions

Table 4.1 Positive health in lifestyle medicine competencies: Physical activity science, assessment, and prescription

Lifestyle medicine competencies	Positive health expansion
Examine the evidence and pathophysiology between physical activity components and health outcomes	Examine the evidence for the impact of physical activity on mental and emotional health outcomes
Describe the benefits of physical activity in preventing or treating disease in special populations, such as healthy older adults, pregnant women, children and adolescents, persons with obesity or disability, cardiovascular disease, diabetes, cancer, disability, and stroke	Describe the benefits of physical activity on mental and emotional health, increasing positive emotions and promoting protective health factors
Integrate key physical activity assessment tools into clinical practice	Integrate assessment of positive experiences and positive emotions the individual associates with physical activities
Integrate evidence from relevant physical activity literature into treatment protocols for management, remission, or reversal in patients with diabetes, cancer, cardiovascular, and cerebrovascular disease	Integrate the evidence from physical activity literature into treatment protocols for improved mental and emotional health outcomes, as well as increasing resilience and positive health

through the upward spiral theory of lifestyle change (Marshall, 2020). Positive emotions and experiences during a physical activity can lead to nonconscious nudges to do the activity again and again (Van Cappellen et al., 2018). Moreover, we can increase our capacity to come up with creative solutions to barriers, such as busy schedules (Fredrickson, 2004). This tailoring of the lifestyle change process, including physical activity, can also work in underserved populations with low socioeconomic status. (Mendoza-Vasconez et al., 2016).

Reflect on your current physical activity habits. What are your personal experiences with making sure you stay physically active? What supportive self-talk and other supports, including positive emotions, have been most effective for your habits? As you write a physical activity prescription, what emotions come up for you? Is this prescription one you are already incorporating in your life and are maintaining? What's your driver? Pay attention to the positive emotions when envisioning this physical activity type and level. What strengths did you use to make meaningful changes and stay on track? If you are struggling to be as physically active as you'd like, embrace your situation with self-compassion.

This honesty with yourself will help you make an authentic connection with the patient and springboard effective coaching from shared humanity with true understanding. As appropriate, briefly share your experiences with the patient when making the prescription. Emphasize what you lean on, e.g. positive visioning and experiences, strengths, social support, meaning and values, that may serve as examples for the patient and become a role model of how to apply positive psychology for the physical activity pillar.

Clinical Practice Tools for Leveraging Positive Psychology to Promote Physical Activity

Positive psychology approaches can be emphasized in the clinical steps for assessing and supporting physical activity (Sarin et al., 2022).

History Taking: When you collect in-depth information from the patient about their current and past physical activity experiences and potential influencers and barriers, you have an excellent opportunity to assess positive facilitators for making behavior changes, especially positive feelings that the patient associates with physical activity.

Screening: You can observe positive personal drivers of physical activity when screening the patient according to the American College of Sports Medicine preparticipation guidelines. Assessing current activity level, patient motivation and readiness to make a change can highlight positive activity experiences. For example, a patient may have had greater success and positive recent or distant memories of engaging in sports than in non-sport activities.

Prescription: You can prescribe a physical activity goal supported with positive psychology according to the FITT framework – frequency, intensity, type, and time. The prescription can be enhanced with positive psychology approaches – by adding the three S's – sharing, strengths, and savoring. The first S is for sharing: With whom can you share this goal? The second S is for strengths: What strengths can you use to help you achieve this goal? The third S is for savoring: pay attention to positive emotional and physical feelings while accomplishing this goal. This kind of prescription sets the stage for change even before coaching, bridging the basic physical activity prescription with powerful positive psychology supports for a successful action plan.

Example: Physical Activity Prescription

Walking [type]
Moderate intensity, in which you can still carry on a conversation while walking [intensity]
Daily [frequency]
15 minutes [time]

Include the three Ss:

- Sharing: Identify someone with whom can you share this goal or do the activity
- Strengths: Use your strengths to help you achieve this goal
- Savoring: Pay attention to positive feelings while doing the activity and accomplishing this goal

REFILLS: Unlimited.

Action Plan: For patients who are ready to make a change, you can help them write an action plan that they are confident they can do at a level of 7 or above (on a scale of 1 – lowest confidence level – to 10 – highest confidence level). Include specific examples for fulfilling the three S's, sharing, strengths, and savoring. The action plan spells out feasible action steps, and emphasizing the three Ss concretely brings attention to factors that can support progress.

Additional Positive Psychology Approaches for Increasing Physical Activity

Positive psychology interventions designed to cultivate positive emotions, such as gratitude, optimism, and happiness, are often simple and easy to perform. They can be integrated into daily life, for example, gratitude journaling, savoring, and mindfulness, to leverage many benefits, including increases in physical activity.

Incorporating such positive activities, in addition to well-known approaches such as positive self-talk and step-wise goal settings, into physical activity interventions may help individuals overcome the challenge of being physically active. The empirical literature shows that these techniques have been applied to a variety of contexts, including sports, education, and healthcare, to promote positive psychological outcomes (Carragher et al., 2016). Health coaches have been early adopters of positive psychology techniques, which are increasingly applied in behavior change programs.

Goal Setting

Goal-setting, the process of identifying specific, measurable, achievable, relevant, and time-bound (SMART) goals to work toward (Locke & Latham, 2019), is commonly used by health coaches. In the context of physical activity, goal-setting may involve increasing the number of steps taken each day, running a certain distance, or attending a certain number of exercise classes per week. By setting SMART goals, individuals can have a clear understanding of what they want to achieve and can track and celebrate their progress – even partial progress – toward their goal which boosts positive, reinforcing emotions.

Research has shown that goal-setting can be an effective strategy to increase physical activity levels. Two randomized controlled trials, one with male Latinos (Larsen et al., 2020) and another with female Latinas (Hartman et al., 2017), found that individuals who received a tailored physical activity intervention that included goal-setting were more likely to meet the recommended levels of physical activity compared to those who received a standard physical activity intervention (Larsen et al., 2020). In addition, individuals who set goals were more likely to maintain their physical activity levels over time. Associating a physical activity goal with a positive vision – a personal outcome that feels particularly meaningful, may drive persistence to achieve and maintain a goal. For example, achieving the goal of walking two miles a day may allow an individual to travel and visit a museum or other special place on their bucket list.

Self-Efficacy

Another positive psychology technique commonly applied in health coaching behaviors, including physical activity is self-efficacy. Self-efficacy refers to an individual's belief in their ability to perform a specific behavior (Bandura, 1997). In the context of physical activity, self-efficacy may involve an individual's belief in their ability to perform a certain exercise or participate in a certain physical activity. This positive belief helps them feel more confident and motivated to engage in physical activity.

One meta-analysis (Rhodes & Dickau, 2013) found that individuals with higher levels of self-efficacy were more likely to be physically active. Interventions for increasing self-efficacy have been associated with increased physical activity levels, including older adults (McAuley et al., 2003).

Mindfulness

Mindfulness (Kabat-Zinn, 2003) in the context of physical activity may involve focusing on bodily sensations or being aware of one's thoughts and emotions while engaging in physical activity. By incorporating mindfulness into physical activity interventions, individuals may be able to better connect with their bodies and experience physical activity in a more positive and enjoyable way, hence promoting the physical activity behavior.

A systemic review of the role of mindfulness in physical activity suggests that mindfulness-based interventions, especially when specific to physical activity, may be effective in promoting the activity, but that more research is needed to establish the effect and identify potential mechanisms (Schneider, 2019). In addition, mindfulness interventions have been shown to be effective in reducing stress and improving mental health outcomes, which may further facilitate positive feelings related to physical activity (Burpee & Langer, 2005).

Positive Self-Talk

Positive self-talk involves using statements to encourage and motivate oneself (Hardy et al., 2012) or reframe a negative thought into a more positive or productive, yet realistic thought. Examples include statements such as "I am strong and capable" or "I enjoy moving my body and feeling energized."

A study (Hardy et al., 2012) that examined the effects of positive self-talk during exercise showed that those who engaged in positive self-talk had higher levels of self-efficacy and were more likely to be physically active compared to those who did not use positive self-talk. Anxiety can be reduced and self-esteem increased through positive self-talk about physical activity, which may further promote positive psychological outcomes, as well as improve physical health outcomes (Van Raalte et al., 2016).

Gratitude

Gratitude has also been shown to promote physical activity. One study found that older adult participants who engaged in a gratitude intervention were more likely to be physically active than those in a control group (Layous et al., 2017).

Self-Compassion

Although we were not able to find self-compassion interventions for increasing physical activity, a significant association between self-compassion and physical activity was found in a systemic review, suggesting this approach may also be considered while further interventional research is conducted. (Wang et al., 2021).

Personal Strengths

Recognizing individuals' personal strengths is one of the pathways for increasing regular physical activity practice. Using one's strengths is intrinsically motivating (Niemiec et al., 2017), meaning that when we use our strengths for physical activity, we are more likely to do it because we want to, not because we have to do it. Also, the use of personal strengths is more meaningful and enjoyable, creating a positive feedback loop with an activity, thus fueling it to keep going. Character strength recognition can help individuals engage their strengths in their physical activity practice. Also, specific strength groups have been recognized as supporting physical activity practice (Moradi et al., 2014).

Specifically, virtues of wisdom and knowledge (curiosity for learning and perspective) and temperance (self-control, prudence, humbleness, and modesty) were associated with exercise frequency. Thus, developing these strengths can potentially help individuals engage in more physical activity.

Character Strengths and Exercise

Complete your character strengths profile (www.viacharacter.org) and use your top five character strengths to enhance your practice. For example, if your strength is social intelligence, opt for exercising with your friends; if it is perseverance, set up more challenging goals for yourself; if it is kindness, focus on ways in which you can be kind to your body when exercising.

Case Study of Positive Health Approaches for Physical Activity

Patient Background: Maria, a 63-year-old black grandmother, was diagnosed with hypertension and type 2 diabetes six months ago. She has been taking antihypertensive and hypoglycemic medications without significant improvement in her blood pressure and blood sugar levels and presents to your lifestyle medicine clinic for a change in therapy. She has a sedentary lifestyle and admits that she has been challenged to follow the diet prescribed for her diabetes. She also reports feeling sad and anxious due to her health conditions.

Assessment: The provider conducts an assessment of Maria's physical activity level and emotional state. Maria is not engaged in physical activity except light housework. She is experiencing sadness, anxiety, and frustration due to her health conditions. She worries about getting sicker and not being able to babysit her two grandchildren.

Treatment Plan: Maria's health care team, consisting of her primary care physician and a health psychologist, recommends physical activity with an emphasis on positive emotions as part of her treatment plan.

Intervention from the Inside Out: The plan to increase her activity level, using an emphasis on positive psychology techniques includes the following:

Physical activity treatment plan: The health psychologist discusses the benefits of physical activity on physical and mental health and suggests strategies to increase her activity level. During the activity, she is encouraged to pay attention to her positive feelings. Maria identifies walking in her neighborhood as an activity she could do regularly and that she would enjoy. She has lived in her neighborhood for 30 years, where she feels comfortable. The health psychologist helps her develop an action plan of walking 20 minutes in the late morning after her chores. Maria feels she can walk three times a week to start and increase gradually to every day of the week. The action plan also incorporates positive psychology techniques, such as savoring, sharing/support, strengths, self-talk, mindfulness, and gratitude practice.

Behavioral activation therapy: The health psychologist applies a cognitive-behavioral therapy technique to help Maria reframe some negative thoughts she has had about exercise. Maria had admitted that she had seen herself as a "nonexerciser." They discuss that perhaps she could reframe this thought to seeing herself as someone who could do short walks and emphasizing the pride she feels in adding this to her routine. She can also harness her strength of kindness to support being physically active and help her achieve her meaningful goal of feeling well enough to take care of her grandchildren. Maria agrees to savor the positive feelings and images that come up as she makes progress with her plan. She also explores activities that she enjoys, such as knitting, which gives her a sense of flow, and could help decrease her frustration and anxiety, opening up more energy for achieving her physical activity plan. These approaches harness the positive psychology techniques of using strengths, sharing, and savoring.

Positive psychology intervention: Gratitude journaling: The health psychologist also suggests that Maria keep a gratitude journal, where she could write down three things that she was grateful for once a week. This activity could help her to focus on the positive aspects of her life and improve her positive emotions. Maria is not sure about committing to journaling, but she is happy to write short notes of gratitude to her children and grandchildren.

Character strengths: Upon being asked what she feels are her personal strengths. Maria shares that her kindness is a strength that family and friends often mention. She agrees to direct that kindness to herself in taking better care of herself.

Social support: The health psychologist recommends that Maria involve her family and friends in her physical activity plan and seek their support in encouraging her, and when possible, walking with her. The psychologist also identifies a local support group for individuals with hypertension and diabetes. Maria shared that she is not ready to join a group, but that she would think about it.

Outcome: After three months, Maria is walking 30 minutes three times a week and, usually once with her grandchildren, knitting twice a week, and writing a note of gratitude to one of her family members weekly. Maria's blood pressure and blood sugar levels decreased, and she reports feeling a little less sad and anxious. She also reports that she is ready to join the support group to make new friends.

Key Take-Aways: The case of Maria demonstrates the importance of linking physical activity and positive emotions as part of medical treatment for chronic health conditions, such as diabetes. Integrating the physical activity interventions with behavioral activation therapy that leverages positive emotions and interventions, such as savoring, strengths, gratitude journaling, and social support, can build the foundation for a successful physical health and mental wellbeing treatment program.

Conclusion

Many individuals struggle to meet the recommended levels of physical activity due to barriers such as lack of time, motivation, and resources. Practicing lifestyle medicine from the inside out, which weaves positive psychology approaches into physical activity prescriptions and coaching can help overcome barriers and increase activity levels with resultant powerful mental and physical health benefits. Paying attention to positive emotions experienced during a physical activity enhances the experience and reinforces the desire to continue or increase the activity (as framed in the upward spiral theory of lifestyle change). At the same time, engaging in positive psychology interventions (PPIs), such as gratitude journaling and self-compassion, and leveraging personal strengths can promote resilience and positive emotions which increase one's energy level and creative problem-solving to address lack of time and resource barriers. Therefore, the integration of positive psychology principles can serve an essential role in garnering successful physical activity outcomes, a key pillar of positive health and wellbeing.

References

Babyak, M., Blumenthal, J. A., & Herman, S., Khatri, P., Doraiswamy, M., Moore, K., Craighead, W. E., Baldewicz, T. T., & Krishnan, K. R. (2000). Exercise treatment for major depression: Maintenance of therapeutic benefit at 10 months. *Psychosom Med, 62*, 633–638. https://doi.org/10.1097/00006842-200009000-00006

Bandura, A. (1997). *Self-efficacy: The exercise of control*. W H Freeman and Company.

Blake, H. (2012). Physical activity and exercise in the treatment of depression. *Front Psychiatry, 3*, 106. https://doi.org/10.3389/fpsyt.2012.00106

Blumenthal, J. A., Babyak, M. A., & Doraiswamy, P. M., Watkins, L., Hoffman, B. M., Barbour, K. A., Waugh, R., Hinderliter, A. & Sherwood, A. (2007). Exercise and pharmacotherapy in the treatment of major depressive disorder. *Psychosom Med, 69*(7), 587–596. https://doi.org/10.1097/PSY.0b013e318148c19a

Burpee, L. C., & Langer, E. (2005). Mindfulness and positive psychological functioning. In C. R. Snyder, & S. J. Lopez (Eds.), *Handbook of positive psychology* (pp. 463–475). Oxford University Press.

Carek, P. J., Laibstain, S. E., & Carek, S. M., (2011). Exercise for the treatment of depression and anxiety. *Int J Psychiatry Med, 41*(1), 15–28. https://doi.org/10.2190/PM.41.1.c

Carragher, M., Golding, L., & Mansfield, M. (2016). A systematic review of positive psychology interventions in sport. *International Review of Sport and Exercise Psychology, 9*(1), 50–63.

Carver, C. S., & Scheier, M. F. (2014). Dispositional optimism. *Trends in Cognitive Sciences, 18*(6), 293–299. https://doi.org/10.1016/j.tics.2014.02.003.

Cekin, R. (2015). Psychological benefits of regular physical activity: Evidence from emerging adults. *Universal Journal of Educational Research, 3*(10), 710–717. https://doi.org/10.13189/ujer.2015.031008.

Chen, R., Rosario, K., Lockman, A., Boehm, J., Bousquet-Santos, K., Siegel, E., Mendes, W. B., & Kubzansky, L. D. (2023). Effects of induced optimism on subjective states, physical activity, and stress reactivity. *Journal of Positive Psychology, 18*(4), 592–605. https://doi.org/10.1080/17439760.2022.2070529.

Cooney, G. M., Dwan, K., & Greig, C. A., Lawlor, D. A., Rimer, J., Waugh, F. R., McCurdo, M., & Mead, G. E. (2013). Exercise for depression, *Cochrane Database Syst Rev, 9*. https://doi.org/10.1002/14651858.CD004366.pub6

Dinas, P. C., Koutedakis, Y., & Flouris, A. D. (2011). Effects of exercise and physical activity. *Ir J Med Sci, 180*, 319–325. https://doi.org/10.1007/s11845-010-0633-9

Ernst, C., Olson, A. K., Pinel, J. P., Lam, R. W., & Christie, B. R. (2006). Antidepressant effects of exercise: Evidence for an adult-neurogenesis hypothesis? *J Psychiat Neurosci, 31*(2), 83–92.

Feig, E. H., Harnedy, L. E., Golden, J., Thorndike, A. N., Huffman, J. C., & Psaros, C. (2022). A qualitative examination of emotional experiences during physical activity post-metabolic/Bariatric surgery. *Obes Surg, 32*(3), 660–670. https://doi.org/10.1007/s11695-021-05807-x.

Fredrickson, B. L. (2004). The broaden-and-build theory of positive emotions. *Phil Trans R Soc Lond, 359*, 1367–1377. https://doi.org/10.1098/rstb.2004.1512

Hallgren, M., Stubbs, B., & Vancampfort, D., Lundinm A., Jääkallio, P, & Forsell, Y. (2017). Treatment guidelines for depression: Greater emphasis on physical activity is needed. *European Psychiatry, 40*, 1–3. https://doi.org/10.1016/j.eurpsy.2016.08.011

Hansen, C. J., Stevens, L. C., & Coast, R. (2001). Exercise duration and mood state: How much is enough to feel better? *Health Psychol, 20*(4), 267–275. https://doi.org/10.1037//0278-6133.20.4.267.

Hardy, J., Hall, C. R., & Hardy, L. (2012). Quantifying athlete self-talk: Development and validation of the sport self-talk questionnaire. *Journal of Sport and Exercise Psychology, 34*(6), 878–897. https://doi.org/10.1080/02640410500130706.

Hartman, S. J., Dunsinger, S. I., & Bock, B. C., Larsen, B. A., Linke, S., Pekmezi, D., Marquez, B., Gans, K. M., Mendoza-Vasconez, A. S., & Marcus, B. H. (2017).

Physical activity maintenance among Spanish-speaking Latina in a randomized controlled trial of an internet-based intervention. *J Behav Med, 40*(3), 392–402. https://doi.org/10.1007/s10865-016-9800-4

Hogan, C. L., Catalino, L. I., & Muta, J., Fredrickson, B. L. (2015). Beyond emotional benefits: Physical activity and sedentary behavior affect psychosocial resources through emotions. *Psychol & Health, 30*(3), 354–369. https://doi.org/10.1080/088 70446.2014.973410

Huffman, J. C., Golden, J., Massey, C. N., Feig, E. H., Chung, W. J., Millstein, R. A., Brown, L., Gianangelo, T., Healy, B. C., Wexler, D. J., Park, E. R., & Celano, C. M. (2021). A positive psychology-motivational interviewing program to promote physical activity in type 2 diabetes: The BEHOLD-16 pilot randomized trial. *General Hospital Psychiatry, 68*, 65–73. https://doi.org/10.1016/j.genhosppsych.2020. 12.001

Kabat-Zinn, J. (2003). Mindfulness-based interventions in context: Past, present, and future. *Clinical Psychology: Science and Practice, 10*(2), 144–156. https://doi.org/ 10.1093/clipsy.bpg016.

Kandola, A., Ashdown-Franks, G., & Hendrikse, J., Sabiston, C. M., & Stubbs, B. (2019). Physical activity and depression: Towards understanding the antidepressant mechanisms of physical activity. *Neurosci BioBehav Rev, 107*, 525–539. https://doi. org/10.1016/j.neubiorev.2019.09.040

Kim, E. S., Kubzansky, L. D., Soo, J., & Boehm, J. K. (2017a). Maintaining healthy behavior: A prospective study of psychological well-being and physical activity. *Ann Behav Med, 51930*, 337–347. https://doi.org/10.1007/s12160-016-9856-y

Kim, J., Lee, S., Chun, S., Han, A., & Heo, J. (2017b). The effects of leisure-time physical activity for optimism, life satisfaction, psychological well-being, and positive affect among older adults with loneliness. *Annals of Leisure Research, 20*(4), 406–415. https://doi.org/10.1080/11745398.2016.1238308.

Koh, Y. S., Asharan, P. V., Devi, F., Roystonn, K., Wang, P., Vaingankar, J. A., Abdin, E., Sum, C. F., Lee, E. S., Müller-Riemenschneider, F., Chiong, S. A., & Subramaniam, M. (2022). A cross-sectional study of the perceived barriers to physical activity and their associations with domain-specific physical activity and sedentary behavior. *BMC Public Health, 22*, 1051. https://doi.org/10.1186/s12889-022-13431-2

Larsen, B. A., Benitez, T. J., & Mendoza-Vasconez, A. S., Hartman, S. J., Linke, S. E., Pekmezi, D. J., Dunsiger, S. I., Nodroa, J. N., Gans, K. M., & Marcus, B. H. (2020). Randomized trial of a physical activity intervention for Latino med: Activo. *Am J Prev Med., 59*(2), 219–227. https://doi.org/10.1016/j.amepre.2020.03.007

Lathia, N., Sandstrom, G. M., Mascolo, C., & Rentfrow, P. J. (2017). Happier people live more active lives: Using smartphones to link happiness and physical activity. *PLoS One, 12*(1), e0160589. https://doi.org/10.1371/journal.pone.0160589.

Layous K, Chancellor J, Lyubomirsky S. (2014) Positive activities as protective factors against mental health conditions. *J Abnorm Psychol. 123*(1):3–12. doi: 10.1037/ a0034709.

Li, J., Huang, Z., Si, W., & Shao, T. (2022). The effects of physical activity on emotions in children and adolescents: A systematic review and meta-analysis. *Int J Environ Res Public Health, 19*(21), 14185. https://doi.org/10.3390/ijerph192114185.

Lianov, L. S., Adamson, K., & Kelly, J. H., Matthews, S., Palma, M., & Rea, B. L. (2022). Lifestyle medicine core competencies: 2022 update. *Am J Lifestyle Med, 16*(6), 734–739. https://doi.org/10.1177/15598276221121580

Locke, E. A., & Latham, G. P. (2019). *New developments in goal-setting and task performance*. Routledge.

Mammen, G., & Faulkner, G. (2013). Physical activity and the prevention of depression: A systematic review of prospective studies. *Am J Prev Med, 45*(5), 649–657. https://doi.org/10.1016/j.amepre.2013.08.001.

Mann, A., & Nanula, B. Positive psychology in sports: An overview. *International Journal of Social Science, 6*(2), 153–158. https://doi.org/10.5958/2321-5771.2017.00017.5

Marshall, D. (2020). The upward spiral of self-development and well-being: An examination of upward spirals and vantage resources and their contribution to sustained self-development, well-being, and lifestyle transformation. Master of Applied Positive Psychology (MAPP) Capstone project. August 1, 2020. https://repository.upenn.edu/server/api/core/bitstreams/d7e4187b-c806-49d2-9577-51ca59f3d47e/content

McAuley, E., Jerome, G. J., Elavsky, S., Marquez, D. X., Ramsey, S. N., & Fruge, A. D. (2003). Predicting long-term maintenance of physical activity in older adults. *Preventive Medicine, 37*(2), 110–118.

McKercher, C., Sanderson, K., & Schmidt, M. D., Otahal, P., Patton, G. C., Dwyer, T., & Venn, A. J. (2014). Physical activity patterns and risk of depression in young adulthood: A 20-year cohort study since childhood. *Soc Psychiatry Psychiatr Epidemiol, 49*(11), 1823–1834.

Mendoza-Vasconez, A. S., Linke, S. E., Munoz, M. A., & Pekmezi, D. (2016). Promoting physical activity among underserved populations. *Curr Sports Med Rep, 15*(4), 290–297. https://doi.org/10.1249/JSR.0000000000000276.

Millstein, R., Golden, J., Healy, B. C., Amonoo, H. L., Harnedy, L. E., Carillo, A., Celano, C. M., & Huffman, J. C. (2022) Latent curve modeling of physicial activity trajectories in a positive-psychology and motivational interviewing intervention for people with type 2 diabetes. *Health Psychol. Behav. Med. 10*(1), 713–730. https://doi.org/10.1080/21642850.2022.2104724

Moradi, S., Nima, A. A., Ricciari, M. R., Archer, T., Garcia, D. (2014). Exercises, character strengths, wellbeing, and learning climate in the prediction of performance over a 6-month period at a call center. *Front Psychol., 5.* https://doi.org/10.3389/fpsyg.2014.00497

Newall, N. E. G., Chipperfield, J. G., Bailis, D. S., & Stewart, T. L. (2012). Consequences of loneliness on physical activity and mortality in older adults and the power of positive emotions. *Health Psychol, 32*(8), 921–924. https://doi.org/10.1037/a0029413.

Niemiec, R. M., Shogren, K. A., & Wehmeyer, M. L. (2017) Character strengths and intellectual and developmental disability: A strengths-based approach from positive psychology. *Education and Training in Autism and Developmental Disabilities, 52*(1), 13–25.

Piercy, K. L., Troiano, R. P., Ballard, R. M., Carlson, S. A., Fulton, J. E., Galuska, D. A., George, S. M., & Olson, R. D. (2018). The physical activity guidelines for Americans. *Journal of the American Medical Association, 320*(19), 2020–2028. https://doi.org/10.1001/jama.2018.14854.

Proyer, R. T., Gander, F., Wellenzohn, S., & Willibald, R. (2013). What good are character strengths beyond subjective wellbeing? The contribution of the good character on self-reported health-oriented behavior, physical fitness, and the subjective health status. *J Pos Psychol, 8*(3), 222–232. https://doi.org/10.1080/17439760.2013.777767.

Rimer, J., Dwan, K., & Lawlor, D. A., Greig, C. A., McCurdo, M., Morley, W., & Mead, G. E. (2012). Exercise for depression, *Cochrane Db Syst Rev, 11*(7). https://doi.org/10.1002/14651858.CD004366.pub6

Rhodes, R. E., & Dickau, L. (2013). Moderators of the intention-behavior relationship in the physical activity domain: A systematic review. *Br J Sports Med, 47*(4), 215–225. https://doi.org/10.1136/bjsports-2011-090411.

Rhodes, R. E., & Kates, K. A. (2015). Can the affective response to exercise predict future motives and physical activity behavior? A systematic review of published evidence. *Ann Behav Med, 49*(5), 715–731. https://doi.org/10.1007/s12160-015-9704-5.

Sarin, S., Motta, M., & Gobble, J. E. (2022). *The practitioner's guide to lifestyle medicine*. Healthy Learning.

Schneider, J., Malinowski, P., Watson, P. M., & Lattimore, P. (2019). The role of mindfulness in physical activity: A systemic review. *Obesity Reviews, 20*(3), 448–463. https://doi.org/10.1111/obr.12795.

Van Cappellen, P., Rice, E. L., & Catalino, L. I., & Fredrickson, B. L. (2018) Positive affective processes underlie positive health behavior change. *Psychol Health, 33*(1), 77–97. https://doi.org/10.1080/08870446.2017.1320798

Van Raalte, J. L., Vincent, A., & Brewer, B. W. (2016). Self-talk: Review and sport-specific model. *Psychology of Sport and Exercise, 22*, 139–148. https://doi.org/10.1016/j.psychsport.2015.08.004

Wang, M. Y. C., Chung, P.-K., & Leung, K.-M. (2021). The relationship between physical activity and self-compassion: A systemic review and meta-analysis. *Mindfulness, 12*, 547–563. https://doi.org/10.1007/s12671-020-01513-4

5 Positive Psychology and Sleep for Positive Health

Chapter Overview

This chapter highlights the science of the reciprocal link between sleep and mood and provides practical guidance for enhancing clinical approaches and coaching applications that use PERMA and other positive psychology interventions to promote sleep health.

Introduction

To gain the physiologic, mental, and emotional health benefits of sleep, the average healthy adult needs seven to seven and a half hours, with a range of seven to nine hours, per night (Watson et al., 2015; Worley, 2018). However, many individuals struggle with sleep disturbances, such as insomnia and sleep deprivation, which can have negative consequences on physical and mental health. Inversely, anxiety, sadness, and other negative emotions can interrupt sleep.

Sleep disturbance is associated with a range of reasons. It may be due to the illness individuals experience (e.g. chronic pain), circumstances (e.g. transatlantic travel), lifestyle (e.g. partying), life stage (e.g. having a young child), or environment (e.g. noisy neighborhood). Each one of the reasons for sleeplessness comes with a range of beliefs that can help or hinder recovery. For example, experiencing jetlag may cause temporary frustration, but we believe we will soon recover once the travel ends. Therefore, we are more likely to take action to remedy this and employ short-term solutions, such as realigning our circadian rhythm to synchronize with the time zone or using sleep aids such as melatonin.

It is different when the sleep disturbance is due to something we cannot easily control. Having a young child may be associated with the belief that we will not get a good night's sleep for a very long time. This, in turn, may lead to feelings of hopelessness and worsening of symptoms leading to

DOI: 10.4324/9781003428909-5

inertia. We choose not to take action, instead, we just brace ourselves and suffer the consequences. Moreover, we may start perceiving ourselves pejoratively, given that so many other people can sustain sleepless nights minding their infants while we cannot. This is why it is crucial to understand what lies beneath the sleep disturbance, to identify beliefs that patients may carry, and which impact their effect.

The Reciprocal Link between Sleep and Emotions

Poor quality or inadequate sleep is associated with negative emotions, such as anger, irritability, and depression, and overall poor psychological wellbeing in a negative reinforcing cycle (Dinges et al., 1997; Lollies et al., 2022; Lopresti et al., 2013; Steptoe et al., 2008; Yoo et al., 2007). Sleeping one-and-a-half to two hours less than usual can lead to these consequences (Saksvik-Lehouillier et al., 2020). At the same time, positive emotions and sleep have a bi-directional relationship (Moskowitz & Saslow, 2014). Good quality sleep is associated with experiencing positive emotions and health, but also experiencing positive emotions before sleep is associated with better quality sleep.

This association may be due to a range of reasons. For example, greater sleep quality predicts daily heart rate variability (HRV); at the same time, HRV has a direct influence on positive emotions (Ballesio et al., 2023). Thus, when we get a good night's sleep, our HRV the next day is higher, which becomes a springboard to experiencing more positive emotions. Also, after a good night's sleep, we are more likely to attend to positive stimuli, such as finding joy in simple daily moments or arranging a meeting with a friend (Gujar et al., 2011). We also tend to have better memory for positive events (Walker & van der Helm, 2009), meaning we can easily recall the good things that have happened in the past, which we can either replicate or allow to impact our present lives. This recall is fundamental for wellbeing, as the happiest people spend significant time each day thinking about the positive past (Boniwell & Zimbardo, 2004). Positive psychology offers a range of interventions that encourage individuals to tap into the positive past perspective. The two boxes offer examples of these interventions.

Positive Reminiscence (Adapted from Bryant et al., 2004)

Begin by writing down several positive memories. Now, select one and over the next ten minutes, sit quietly, take a few deep breaths, close your eyes (if it is safe to do so) and think intensely about this memory. See the images your mind is creating, feel the emotions your memory elicits, and bask in the joy of re-experiencing your past.

Intensely Positive Experiences (Adapted from Burton & King, 2004)

Consider some of your life's happiest, most joyful, life-affirming moments. This could be your child's birth, being moved by music or a piece of art, or seeing a sunset over the mountains. Now, select one memory, and for the next 15–20 minutes, write, in as much detail as you can master, about your experience. Focus on your thoughts, feelings, emotions, and all the circumstances surrounding your positive memory. Enjoy re-experiencing it.

After a good night's sleep, the positive reminiscence activities associated with the richness of positive memories are much easier to access. However, they can also help us improve our positive emotions before sleep. What is important is that we choose an activity best suitable for us, an activity we enjoy. These may include interventions such as reading a book before bed, listening to favorite music, or doing breathing exercises (Burke et al., 2022). Another effective way to improve sleep is by unplugging our digital devices.

Our experiment asked participants to leave their phones behind for one hour before sleep for one week (Hughes & Burke, 2018). When forced not to use digital devices, many participants initially panicked. They wondered what they would do for the last hour before bed. After all, so many of us tend to use our phones last thing at night and first thing in the morning. However, many of them were surprised by the effect after accepting this challenge. Turning off their devices allowed them to spend more time preparing for the next day, reflecting on the day just gone, do other things they used to do in bed, such as reading a book. Many have also noted that they spent more time with their partners, talking to them, cuddling, and having sex. Finally, by the end of this week's experiment, over 90% of participants were willing to continue with it. Apart from changing pre-sleeping habits, this experiment resulted in increased wellbeing and improvement in the quality of sleep. This is just one example of how a simple action can spark positive change.

Sleep is associated with mood. Moods differ from emotions in that they are at a more subconscious level, free-floating and not necessarily associated with specific stimuli. Positive emotions, on the other hand, are often associated with a specific event or circumstance (Fredrickson & Losada, 2005). In a study conducted by the University of Pennsylvania, participants limited to four and a half hours of sleep per night for one week reported feeling more stressed, angry, sad, and mentally exhausted (Dinges et al., 1997). However, significant improvement in mood was reported after they returned to their usual longer sleep patterns. This experiment demonstrated the adverse impact of even short-term sleep disruption, but also the resilience of our bodies which are able to recover so promptly afterwards.

One's mood at wake time is also associated with mood before sleep and dream positivity bias (Barbeau et al., 2022). When participants of this study were asked to describe their mood before sleep, mood after sleep, and the dreams they had, those who were effectively processing adverse events and associated with their emotions during sleep tended to rate their emotions more positively than they were objectively rated by an external person (positivity bias). This, in turn, allowed them to experience an improved mood in the morning. Thus, one's mood may improve either after a good night's sleep or due to developing effective strategies that allow one to process negative emotions.

Another way to improve mood is via accumulated positive emotions that build psychological and intellectual resources (Fredrickson, 2004). Equally, experiencing many negative emotions is associated with poorer sleep outcomes. For example, insomnia patients reported higher levels of negative emotions and, subsequently, more negative dream content than individuals who do not experience insomnia (Pérusse et al., 2016). Hence, the emotions that individuals experience and the associated thoughts play a significant role in sleep.

Positive psychology techniques, such as gratitude, mindfulness, cognitive-behavioral therapy (CBT), and satisfying, meaningful activities, that lead to increased positive emotions may be effective in promoting better sleep quality and overall sleep health. Empirical studies suggest both positive affect and eudaimonic wellbeing – a life with meaning and purpose – are shown to be associated with good sleep (Steptoe et al., 2008). This means that by helping patients increase their experiences of positive emotions and building foundations for living a good life, their sleep quality may improve. However, empirical data is limited, and more high-quality research is needed (Ong et al., 2017).

Life Purpose and Sleep Health

Whilst sleep is impacted by and impacts the experiences of emotions, other positive psychological processes, such as having a life purpose, also influence it. Life purpose is the expression of life's meaning. Meaning in life is a theoretical exploration of what matters to us, whereas life purpose is the application of our meaning (Burke, 2021) and a motivational force to realize it (Steger, 2017). For example, my meaning in life may be to make people healthier and happier. I aim to spread the word about positive psychology research to help others use it more effectively (my life purpose). Therefore, a life purpose is what we do with what we value and find worthwhile.

Life purpose has been associated with sleep across many studies. For example, individuals with a well-carved purpose in life demonstrate less body movement during sleep, which in turn helps them improve their sleep quality (Ryff et al., 2004). Also, those who experienced sleep disturbance, such as too much or inadequate sleep, tended to have lower levels of life purpose

(Hamilton et al., 2007). These findings may also be associated with meaning, given that purpose is an expression of it. Research shows that while the presence of meaning in life is a foundation for a good life, physical health and wellbeing (Roepke et al., 2014; Steger, 2017), searching for life meaning is associated with an inverse effect (Li et al., 2021).

Furthermore, individuals pursue goals they value when they have a life purpose. Human beings are intrinsically goal-oriented. Our ultimate goal is survival. Goal-less lives are unhappy lives as we cannot consciously grow, monitor our progress, or practice our self-confidence without having goals. Depressed individuals tend to have fewer goals than non-depressed; they do not believe they can accomplish their goals and tend to focus on avoiding bad situations rather than striving toward better ones (Dickson et al., 2016). Given that life purpose is closely related to goal-striving, it becomes clearer why those who do not have a clearly defined life purpose may be more likely to experience sleep disturbance.

At the same time, a cross-sectional study with British civil servants demonstrated that after controlling for demographics, such as age or gender, individuals with higher levels of self-reported purpose reported better sleep outcomes (Steptoe et al., 2008). Similarly, a longitudinal study exploring the impact of sleep over time showed that purpose in life was a protective factor against developing sleeping problems (Phelan et al., 2010). Whilst, on average, participants' sleep quality declined over a decade, those with higher levels of psychological wellbeing, including having a life purpose, showed a slower decline and fewer sleep disturbances. Thus, purpose in life plays an important role in sleep.

Several interventions have been developed to assist individuals in exploring their life meaning and purpose. Their objective is to provide space for people to think through what is important in their lives (meaning) and then come up with small steps toward realizing their meaning (purpose). We offer a suggestion in the box.

Life Crafting (Adapted from Schippers & Ziegler, 2019)

Every day, over the next few days, spend 15–20 minutes exploring the following:

- What is important to you? What are your values and passions in life?
- What are you good at?
- How satisfied are you with your social life? What else can you do to become more satisfied?
- If all went well, what would you like to accomplish in your personal and career life?

Write about your ideal future in the context of these questions. In your writing, include goals that will help you realize your ideal future, and what obstacles might get in the way of it happening. For each obstacle, come up with an action plan on what you will do when they happen. Finally, share your goals with your family and friends.

Optimism and Sleep Health

Optimism is an expectation that all in life will work out well. Many theories of optimism exist. Dispositional optimism is a trait and state of optimism (Kluemper et al., 2009). It is perceived as a predisposition to expect the best in the future and a temporary feeling of optimism. On the other hand, the explanation style significantly emphasizes individuals' thoughts (Seligman, 2006). According to this theory, people are not necessarily pessimistic or optimistic; instead, they think pessimistic and optimistic thoughts. As such, they can control their thinking and subsequent outcomes by choosing a more optimistic style.

When something terrible happens to a person who practices pessimistic thinking, they may, firstly, blame their stable characteristics (e.g. IQ, personality) for it, thus making it less likely for them to take action and change. On the other hand, optimistic thinkers may partially hold themselves responsible for the negative outcome. However, they will also be able to see the bigger picture, i.e. consider the circumstances and other people involved. As such, they will say, "I made a mistake at work because I was not careful," or "there were many distractions today, and I did not get a good night's sleep." All these reasons do not "attack" them as people, but rather what they did, which can be changed. This thinking is very different from saying, "I am such a dummy! I am no good as a doctor." Pessimistic thinking makes us passive and unable to resolve the situation, whereas optimistic thinking allows us to find a motivation to change our circumstances, behaviors, and attitudes and keep going.

Secondly, people who think pessimistically perceive their bad luck or adverse outcomes as lasting forever. When they make a mistake, they say things like: "They will never let me forget" or "This will never change." On the other hand, optimistic thinkers will create time restrictions for their mistakes and bad things happening to them. They will say: "It is temporary. This too shall pass," or "I will find a way to change their mind about me." This type of thinking allows individuals to take action and reverse the dire situation. At the same time, pessimistic thinking that something will last for a long time will make them less likely to take action.

Thirdly, when a bad thing happens to pessimistic thinkers, they tend to say that "everything" is terrible. They see a connection between their adverse event and all their aspects of life. "I made a mistake," they say, "now my life is ruined." Optimistic thinkers, on the other hand, can compartmentalize their lives. They say, "Fine, I have made a mistake in my diagnosis, but I am usually good at my job," or "My job is not going very well at the moment, but at least my personal life is good, and I have some vacation that will help me relax." By separating the adverse event from other aspects of their lives, optimistic thinkers can step back and change their perspective, which ultimately helps them take action.

Optimism is necessary for survival, as it helps us keep going regardless of circumstances. It is no wonder that neuropsychological studies found that most people are optimistic (Sharot, 2011). At the same time, when pessimistic, people are at high risk of developing depression (Garrett & Sharot, 2017) and experiencing a lower quality of sleep (Uchino et al., 2017). This is why, in a cross-sectional study with over 1,000 people, optimistic people were at a significantly lower risk of experiencing insomnia than pessimists (Weitzer et al., 2021). In this study, optimism was a better predictor of good sleep than lifestyle choices. Thus, exploring interventions that aim to help patients change their thinking style to be more optimistic may become a future approach for insomnia. A cognitive behavioral therapy approach is applied to help people do it (Seligman, 2006). Positive health coaches trained to explore optimistic and pessimistic thinking may also assist patients in doing it.

Post-Traumatic Growth (PTG) to Support Sleep after Trauma

PTG refers to psychological growth after experiencing trauma. Over 70% of individuals experience PTG in at least one domain (Joseph, 2013). It is a natural process that occurs to help us cope with adversity. According to Tedeschi and Calhoun (2004), the five domains within which growth occurs relate:

1 Personal strengths or changes within self – individuals see themselves post-trauma as stronger than they thought they were, more confident, mature, and alive.
2 Relating to others – an individual reports being closer to some people, becoming tighter with family members or friends.
3 Appreciation for life – an individual becomes aware of how short life is and starts considering topics such as mortality, meaning in life, and purpose.
4 New possibilities – an individual begins to see opportunities for change, learning new skills, enrolling in an educational institution, and changing their life goals.
5 Spirituality – an individual becomes more spiritual, closer to God or a higher being.

PTG realization is an essential process for coping with trauma. For example, in a study with childless women, we found that after controlling for longing to have a child, experiencing PTG predicted participants' high psychological, emotional, and social wellbeing levels (Burke & Meehan, 2023). The two PTG domains that seemed to protect childless women's wellbeing were seeing new possibilities in their lives without children and relating to others.

PTG can also occur in healthcare professionals, many of whom experience trauma in their work or personal lives. Recently, we conducted a systematic review of PTG research in healthcare and identified various factors that support healthcare professionals in experiencing PTG (O'Donovan & Burke, 2022). They ranged from the work environment conditions (e.g. workload, patient population, interpersonal factors, relational support at work), interventions used and individual factors such as perceived meaning for work or levels of self-compassion. Thus, a range of factors beyond the traumatic event facilitates growth.

Please note that Joseph (2013) warned against setting up an objective for PTG, as it is an outcome of the traumatic process that happens naturally. Some questions and reflections can facilitate PTG, making us more likely to experience it. But the process should not be forced. Positive psychology interventions can support patients in facilitating their experiences of growth post-trauma and help alleviate sleep disturbances associated with trauma.

For example, 40 patients who had experienced renal transplantation underwent a four-week psychotherapeutic program based on positive psychology (Látos et al., 2022).

- In week 1, the objective of the week was to increase positive emotions by discussing the negative emotions associated with the transplant and then drawing patients' attention to the positive emotions that they have also experienced, e.g. gratitude for being able to make the surgery, love for their family and friends who supported them, the micro-moments of fun and laughter with the doctors.
- In week 2, the therapists focused on creating meaning for patients, accepting their sickness, and making a new meaning to their life post-recovery.
- In week 3, the stability of their body and boundaries are discussed, and the therapist focuses on the patient's capabilities and what they can do rather than what they cannot.
- In week 4, an optimistic thinking style is practiced to help patients develop positive expectations about their lives ahead.

The positive psychology interventions practiced during those four weeks related to savoring the moment, gratitude, kindness, empathy, optimism, and strength and meaning-making. Following the four-week intervention, patients' PTG scores increased significantly and were higher than the control group's.

Furthermore, the patient's estimated glomerular filtration rate and serum creatinine levels were significantly improved among patients receiving positive psychology intervention at 6- and 12-month follow-ups. While sleep was not measured in this study, it provides an example of how PTG can be experienced by patients undergoing positive psychology interventions. Given that PTG is associated with better sleep (Sheikh-Wu et al., 2023), further research needs to explore it in the context of various patient populations.

Practical Applications of Positive Psychology for Sleep Health

Positive psychology can be applied in practical ways by health practitioners to promote sleep hygiene, along with emotional and mental health, leading to physical benefits reinforced by other lifestyle pillars that can result in positive health.

PERMA and Sleep Health

The PERMA framework can be used to guide questions that prompt the individual to discover and create ways to increase positive emotions for improved sleep hygiene habits and achieving restorative sleep. The list below offers suggested questions to harness PERMA for promoting sleep health.

Application of PERMA to Promote Sleep Health

P—Positive emotions: Pay attention to the positive aspects of your day and your life. Reflect on these experiences before bedtime.
- When have you experienced calming and positive feelings at bedtime?
- What kinds of thoughts and activities bring forth feelings of calm and positivity for you?
- How can you increase positive experiences throughout the day, and especially at the end of the day before getting ready to sleep?

E—Engagement (Flow): Do activities that put you in a state of flow, a state of mindfulness when your thoughts are directed to an activity, and you forget about time and your surroundings. Doing a flow activity in the evening may calm you from the stress of the day; set an alarm for an hour or two before bedtime in case you lose track of time during the activity.
- What activities have you done in the past or recently that give you a sense of flow?
- What activities can you do in the evenings to help you experience flow and let go of worries?

R—Relationships: Identify how you can increase positive social interactions.
- What are happy or calming activities you can do in the evening and at bedtime that involve others, such as meaningful activities with loved ones?
- What people can you involve in evening routines that relax you and increase positive emotions?

M—Meaning: Pay attention to getting restorative sleep with your values and what is meaningful, such as taking care of yourself to have the energy to complete family commitments.
- What are meaningful ways you can support yourself in following through with a sleep hygiene plan?
- How does achieving a sleep hygiene plan align with your values?
- What daily activities can you recall in the evenings that give you a sense of purpose or feel meaningful?

A—Achievement: At bedtime, reflect on your accomplishments of the day.
- What daily activities can you recall in the evening that give you a sense of accomplishment and pride?
- For those with a sleep hygiene plan (such as avoiding blue screens in the bedroom): what have you achieved in your sleep hygiene plan? If you were not able to achieve your sleep goals, embrace self-compassionate self-talk; take pride in even the smallest successes and efforts.

Appreciative Inquiry to Support Sleep Health

Exploring and developing positive solutions through the appreciative inquiry process can be adapted to support individuals with all of their lifestyle goals, including sleep health. The questions build positive emotions prompted by attention to what is going well now in the context of their sleep health, envisioning possibilities for positive future changes, and determining a plan that uses strengths for increasing self-efficacy.

Discovery: What is good now about your sleep habits?
- What positive experiences and emotions do you recall on nights when you get seven to nine hours of restorative sleep?
- What has been your routine on the nights when you get restorative sleep?
- What sleep hygiene pattern (e.g. lighting and temperature of the bedroom, use of devices and eating habits in the evening) do you associate with your best sleep and your best self?

Dream: What are possible ways to create a healthy sleep hygiene routine?
- What healthy activities could be done that lead to relaxation in the evenings and better sleep health?
- What personal strengths could be used to achieve and maintain nightly restorative sleep?

Design: What changes could you make to build a healthy sleep routine?
- How can you increase or add relaxing activities to your bedtime routine?
- Which of your strengths can you use to achieve better sleep health?
- With whom could you connect to support your goal?

Destiny: What changes are you confident you can make for your healthy sleep action plan?
- What steps will take toward a healthy sleep hygiene routine?
- Which strengths will you use to achieve this action plan?
- What are healthy ways you can reward yourself for achieving your action plan?

Integrating Positive Health into Lifestyle Medicine Competencies for Sleep Health Science and Interventions

Lifestyle medicine competencies in the sleep health science and interventions section can be expanded and enhanced through the lens of positive health.

- When describing sleep's role in health and chronic disease pathophysiology, include how sleep can promote emotional wellbeing, resilience, and thriving, in addition to physical and mental health.
- When performing sleep assessments to identify patients with insufficient or poor-quality sleep, also assess for good sleep hygiene and praise patients who consistently get an adequate amount of restorative sleep. Also, monitor for partial success with sleep goal goals.
- When summarizing lifestyle-based interventions that can improve sleep health, include interventions that increase positive emotions about sleep, techniques that reframe self-talk about sleep, and sleep hygiene approaches that leverage the individual's strengths.

Table 5.1 presents the lifestyle medicine competencies in the area of sleep health in the left column and suggests in the right column an expansion of these competencies for positive health in clinical practice.

Table 5.1 Integrating positive health in lifestyle medicine competencies: Sleep health science and interventions

Lifestyle medicine competency	Positive health expansion
Describe sleep's role in health and chronic disease pathophysiology	Describe how sleep can promote emotional wellbeing, resilience, and thriving, in addition to mental and physical health
Perform sleep assessments to identify patients with insufficient or poor-quality sleep	Assess for and praise healthy sleep hygiene in patients who get restorative sleep consistently; identify and praise partial successes with good sleep hygiene in those who generally get insufficient or poor-quality sleep
Summarize lifestyle-based interventions that can improve sleep health	Summarize interventions that increase positive emotions about sleep, cognitive techniques that reframe self-talk about sleep, and sleep hygiene approaches that harness the individual's strengths

Perspectives on Practicing Lifestyle Medicine from the Inside Out – Sleep Health

Supporting sleep health requires a person-centered, whole health and positive health approach, including investigating the individual's personal historical and environmental factors that affect their sleep habits. Gaining a sense of the individual's cultural views on sleep is also important.

If, for example, as may be the case for many physicians, the individual has a sense that the culture expects them to de-prioritize sleep, an open discussion about that culture and how it affects personal sleep habits and goals is essential. Physicians have been traditionally expected to sacrifice their sleep and be available to take care of their patients, as needed, even in the middle of the night. From a positive psychology perspective, the provider can ask when they have had a positive experience with someone in their environment praising them for taking care of themselves. Examples of questions based on cognitive behavioral and positive psychology techniques that can help shape sleep interventions include:

- What experiences have you had that affect your view of rest and sleep and have shaped your sleep habits? What positive experiences related to sleep have you had?
- How does your community – work, school, family – view sleep? What are acceptable sleep habits in your community? What elements of your community and environment support rest and sleep health?

- How do you see the role of sleep in your health and life? What are your beliefs about the importance of sleep? What positive beliefs can help your sleep health goals?
- How can you reframe your self-talk about sleep to support your sleep health goals?

Past traumas, including post-traumatic stress disorder, can interfere with sleep due to feelings of guilt, anxiety and stress and nightmares, along with many other factors such as medication side effects, pain, and medical and sleep disorders (Sarin et al., 2022). When history taking and screening identify emotions as one of the possible causes, counseling and developing a plan to alleviate these emotions is needed. Discussions about barriers and solutions to restorative sleep can be grounded in positive psychology. Asking questions about positive experiences and memories of when the individual was able to face and resolve difficult situations may counter some sources of stress and anxiety that interfere with sleep.

Helping individuals build awareness about how they have leveraged their strengths in difficult times can also pave the way for positive reflections and self-talk at bedtime. Cognitive reframing (self-talk about what is going well and what they can do to address adversities) and positive reminiscence (recalling good experiences) are empowering skills. Noticing the good along with the bad can serve as an essential tool when they find their mind racing at bedtime or in the middle of the night.

Positive Psychology for Promoting Sleep Health

Positive psychology approaches can be emphasized in the clinical steps for assessing and supporting sleep health (Frates et al., 2020; Sarin et al., 2022). In a study with colorectal cancer survivors, activities relating to PTG and benefit finding have eased the severity of their symptoms, such as pain, dizziness, drowsiness, and sleep disturbance (Sheikh-Wu et al., 2023). In the boxes, we provide an examples of interventions that can be used for benefit-finding.

Benefit-Finding (Adapted from King & Miner, 2000)

Take a piece of paper and, every day for a week, write down for 15–20 minutes the answers to these questions when considering an event or experience.

1 How has this experience benefitted you as a person?
2 How has this event made you better equipped to cope with challenges in the future?

One Door Closes... (Adapted from Gander et al., 2013)

Every day for the next week, reflect on the time in your life when an adverse event occurred and how it caused one door to close for you. Then, consider what happened afterward. What opportunities has this event opened up for you? What have you realized about yourself and others following this adverse event? You can write down your answers or discuss them with a family member or a friend.

The Positive Health Clinical Practice Approach for Sleep Health

History Taking: When assessing for factors that affect sleep, including prescription medications, (e.g. diuretics, steroids, stimulants, over-the-counter (OTC) medications that contain caffeine, alcohol, menopause, and illnesses such as asthma, chronic obstructive pulmonary disease) the provider needs to be on the lookout for psychiatric and psychological conditions (e.g. depression and marital conflicts). During this assessment ask about activities that the patient has noticed can counter the sleep issues and how they have been able to make progress with sleep health currently or in the past. How have they been able to calm themselves or improve their mood to help them sleep? These examples can serve as a springboard for positive health expansion of a sleep health action plan.

Assessment: Assessment for sleep health may involve sleep diaries, wearable devices and apps, and sleep studies. As the provider has much to consider in evaluating the patient for sleep health, it may be easy to overlook what positive actions have taken and what small successes have occurred. These "actions" might involve self-talk and emotional self-soothing methods. Inquiring about and highlighting successes is an important element of the positive psychology approach.

Treatment and Interventions: Besides changing medications and offering treatment for medical and mental illnesses, conditions and lifestyle factors that may be interfering with sleep, e.g. adjusting light exposure and sleep environment, setting routine sleep and wake times, decreasing heavy evening meals, and relaxation exercises before bedtime, the provider can emphasize positive health techniques. Among these is cognitive behavioral therapy which has long been a staple of psychological treatments for insomnia (Frates et al., 2020; Sarin et al., 2022). The intervention prescription can be enhanced with positive psychology constructs like the three S's, sharing the activity or goal with others for social support, using strengths to fulfill the goal, and savoring the positive experiences during and afterward as a consequence of the changes made. This kind of prescription facilitates incorporating such constructs into the action plan.

Prescription: Often the sleep health prescription may start with sleep hygiene education that includes a list of basic action steps, such as going to bed and waking up at the same time, avoiding naps too close to bedtime, and eliminating alcohol. Also, a sleep diary is useful in an evolving process to identify and treat the root of the sleep issue. When a specific problem is identified, a more traditional prescription can be made, e.g. eliminate caffeine for one month as a trial treatment. Then questions to prompt solutions for follow-through and support can be added. With whom can you share this goal? What strengths can you use to help you achieve this goal? Pay attention to positive emotional and physical feelings while accomplishing this goal.

Action Plan: With the help of someone on the health team, the patient can write an action plan that they are confident they can do at a level of 7 or above (on a scale of 1 – lowest confidence level – to 10 – highest confidence level), along with specific steps for sharing, strengths and savoring that bring attention to positive psychology factors for making progress.

Sleep Health Prescriptions

A sleep hygiene prescription can include prompts for the three Ss – sharing, strengths, and savoring – to support the goal. The health coach can then guide the development of an action plan to include these elements and other positive emotion boosters. Examples can be found in the boxes,

---

Example 1: Positive Psychology-Based Sleep Health Prescription – Devices

Retire to the bedroom without devices at least one hour before bedtime
    [type]
Nightly [frequency]
Support this goal with the three Ss:

- Sharing: Identify someone with whom you can share this goal, someone who may also want to eliminate devices at bedtime, or someone who can encourage you in your goal
- Strengths: Use your strengths to help you achieve this goal
- Savoring: Pay attention to positive feelings as you accomplish this goal. When you celebrate steps toward your goal, let those feelings linger.

Example 1: Action Plan

"I will not bring my laptop and phone into the bedroom and turn in around 9 PM. I will keep them charging in the living room every night. I will ask my wife to remind me. My character strength of perseverance will help me. If I slip back to my old habits of using them in bed and she forgets to remind me, I will reaffirm my goal and persevere until I achieve this goal. I will savor the opportunity to relax away from email and bad news in the late evenings, turn to some relaxing music, and reflect on a positive memory or accomplishment that happened during the day."

Example 2: Positive-Psychology-Based Sleep Health Prescription – Caffeine

Eliminate food and drinks that contain caffeine.

Support this goal with the three S's:

- Sharing: Identify someone with whom can you share this goal, someone who may also want to eliminate caffeine or someone who can encourage you in your goal
- Strengths: Use your strengths to help you achieve this goal
- Savoring: Pay attention to positive feelings as you accomplish this goal

Example 2: Action Plan

The patient may be ready, as a first step, to replace their favorite caffeinated drinks with decaffeinated drinks, although the latter may still contain some caffeine. Action Plan: "I will replace my morning coffee and evening tea with decaffeinated alternatives at least 5 days a week. I will ask my sister to remind and encourage me and keep me accountable for this goal. My honesty character strength will help me be honest with her about my progress. I will savor the good feeling that I am doing something to help me sleep better and look for how refreshed I feel as I build my sleep health."

Specific Positive Psychology Interventions
for Sleep Health

As with other lifestyle medicine pillars, a number of positive psychology interventions, such as gratitude practice, mindfulness, and CBT – can be used to improve sleep health. Moreover, other health pillars can contribute to sleep health; physical activity has been especially effective in promoting sleep in individuals with various sleep disorders (Kredlow et al., 2015).

Research has shown that gratitude can be effective in improving sleep quality and duration. A cross-sectional study found that gratitude increased pre-sleep positive cognitions and less negative ones, predicting greater subjective sleep quality and sleep duration (Wood et al., 2009). Another cross-sectional study suggests that gratitude has a modest effect on depression and a stronger effect on anxiety in individuals with chronic pain (Ng & Wong, 2012). The well-known and highly cited study conducted by Emmons and McCullough (2003) found that individuals who kept a daily gratitude journal reported better sleep quality compared to those who kept a daily hassles journal. A systemic review concluded that, although gratitude improved subjective sleep quality in more than half of the studies reviewed and that provided this measure, more research is needed about the impact of gratitude interventions on sleep health outcomes (Boggiss et al., 2020).

Mindfulness, which involves being present at the moment and non-judgmentally observing one's thoughts and feelings, can be effective in sleep health. The process involves focusing on the sensations of the body and breathing during relaxation exercises or being aware of one's thoughts and emotions while falling asleep. A randomized controlled trial (Ong et al., 2012) found that a mindfulness-based intervention was effective in improving sleep quality and reducing insomnia symptoms among older adults. Moreover, another meta-analysis (Gong et al., 2016) found that mindfulness interventions were effective in improving sleep quality among individuals with various sleep disorders.

In a randomized controlled trial that involved a multicomponent intervention, participants were asked to engage in online self-directed training and daily activities that combined mindfulness with a range of wellbeing interventions (Michel et al., 2021). These included brief (2–3 minutes) mindful breathing exercises carried out at work, naming one positive experience that occurred to them at work, practicing an "act of kindness" on a colleague, writing a letter of gratitude to a colleague at work, identifying their character strengths relating to work, or writing about the best future self. These activities performed over three weeks became easily integrated into the work. They resulted in an increase in work engagement and hope for the future. More importantly, they reduced fatigue and increased employees' sleep quality compared to the control group. Given that work is often a reason for many people's sleepless nights, as part of occupational health, these types of interventions can be easily introduced to support them.

CBT for insomnia typically involves identifying and changing negative thought patterns and behaviors that contribute to sleep disturbances. For example, individuals may be taught strategies to manage stress and anxiety, establish a regular sleep schedule, and practice relaxation techniques. One meta-analysis (Smith et al., 2002) found that CBT was effective in improving sleep quality and reducing sleep latency among individuals with chronic insomnia. This benefit of CBT has also been observed in a randomized controlled trial (Espie et al., 2014) among older adults.

Case Study of a Positive Health Approach for Sleep Health

Patient Background: Mary is a 38-year-old single woman (currently without a partner) who works as a teacher and has been coming to the clinic for the management of her inflammatory bowel disease. Although her abdominal pain and diarrhea are less frequent at night, even on nights when her symptoms are minimal, she has had difficulty falling asleep and staying asleep. She often delays going to bed, in anticipation of another bad night. She has tried various OTC sleep medications and sleep aid digital apps, but they have not been effective in improving her sleep duration or quality.

Assessment: A sleep assessment including a review of her medications and habits, is conducted, which suggests that the OTC medication for her pain contains caffeine and also that she has been worried lately about losing her job.

Positive Psychology Intervention: In addition to recommending she stop the OTC that contains caffeine, the provider prescribes a change in her sleep hygiene routine to go to bed at the same time each night. Also, the provider recommends that each evening she take a few minutes to reflect on the positive aspects of her life, such as her supportive friendships and relationships and her fun gardening hobby, and to reframe thoughts about her job worries. The nurse coach teaches Mary techniques for cultivating positive emotions through positive reminiscence, avoiding negative news/reading good news stories, and gratitude journaling.

Outcome: Mary returns in a month and reports she has been jotting down things for which she is grateful about twice a week. She has also been working on redirecting her thoughts away from her worries to thoughts about how her garden has been blooming and the positive comments from neighbors. Although her abdominal pain continues to be an issue some nights, she has been sleeping better overall. She has also been making an effort to seek out good news and listen to relaxing music in the evenings. She feels less anxious at night, has been able to fall asleep more easily, and feels more energized and motivated during the day.

Take-Aways: By focusing on positive emotions and aspects of life, individuals may be able to reduce stress and anxiety that commonly contribute to sleep problems. Positive psychology techniques can be used in conjunction with other sleep hygiene strategies, such as limiting screen time before bed, creating a relaxing bedtime routine, and avoiding caffeine and alcohol before bedtime, to promote healthy sleep habits.

Conclusion

Sleep is an essential healthy lifestyle pillar for positive health. However, many individuals struggle with sleep disturbances, such as insomnia and sleep deprivation. Positive psychology techniques can be integrated into sleep health prescriptions and coaching. The PERMA model and appreciative inquiry can be honed to support sleep hygiene assessment and intervention. Specific PPIs and lifestyle factors, including gratitude, mindfulness, and CBT, and lifestyle habits, especially physical activity, have been shown to be effective in promoting sleep quality. By incorporating these techniques into sleep interventions that address the wide spectrum of factors that interfere with sleep health and by encouraging individuals to use positive psychology in self-care, often restorative sleep can be increased so that its many benefits can be enjoyed as part of positive health.

References

Ballesio, A., Zagaria, A., Salaris, A., Terrasi, M., Lombardo, C., & Ottaviani, C. (2023). Sleep and daily positive emotions—Is heart rate variability a mediator? *Journal of Psychophysiology*, *37*(3), 134–142. https://doi.org/10.1027/0269-8803/a000315

Barbeau, K., Turpin, C., Lafreniere, A., Campbell, E., De Koninck, J. (2022). Dreamers' evaluation of the emotional variance of their day-to-day dreams is indicative of some mood regulation function. *Frontiers in Behavioral Neuroscience*. 16:947396. https://doi.org/10.3389/fnbeh.2022.947396.

Boggiss, A. J., Consedine, N. S., Brenton-Peters, J. S., Hofman, P. L., & Serlachus, A. S. (2020) A systematic review of gratitude interventions: Effects on physical health and health behaviors. *J Psychosom Res.*, *135*, 110165. https://doi.org/10.3389/fnbeh.2022.947396

Boniwell, I., & Zimbardo, P. G. (2004). Balancing time perspective in pursuit of optimal functioning. In P. A. Linley, & S. Joseph (Eds.), *Positive psychology in practice* (pp. 165–178). John Wiley and Sons, Inc.

Bryant, P. A., Trinder, J., & Curtis, N. (2004). Sick and tired: Does sleep have a vital role in the immune system? Nature reviews. *Immunology*, 4(6), 457–467. https://doi.org/10.1038/nri1369

Burke, J. (2021). *The ultimate guide to implementing wellbeing programmes for school.* Routledge.

Burke, J., Dunne, P., Meehan, T., O'Boyle, C., & van Nieuwerburgh, C. (2022). *Positive health: 100+ research-based positive psychology and lifestyle medicine tools to enhance your wellbeing.* Routledge.

Burke, J., & Meehan, T. (2023). Childlessness as a springboard for post-traumatic growth. *Irish Journal of Counselling and Psychotherapy*, 23(1), 4–9.

Burton, C. M., & King, L. A. (2004). The health benefits of writing about intensely positive experiences. *Journal of Research in Personality*, 38(2), 150–163. https://doi-org.elib.tcd.ie/10.1016/S0092-6566(03)00058-8

Dickson, J. M., Moberly, N. J., O'Dea, C., & Field, M. (2016). Goal fluency, pessimism and disengagement in depression. *PLoS One*, 11(11), e0166259. https://doi.org//10.1371/journal.pone.0166259

Dinges, D. F., Pack, F., Williams, K., Gillen, K. A., Powell, J. W., Ott, G. E., Aptowicz, C., & Pack, A. I. (1997). Cumulative sleepiness, mood disturbance, and psychomotor vigilance performance decrements during a week of sleep restricted to 4-5 hours per night. *Sleep*, 20(4), 267–277.

Emmons, R. A., & McCullough, M. E. (2003). Counting blessings versus burdens: An experimental investigation of gratitude and subjective well-being in daily life. *Journal of Personality and Social Psychology*, 84(2), 377–389. https://doi.org/10.1037/0022-3514.84.2.377

Espie, C. A., Kyle, S. D., Williams, C., Ong, J. C., Douglas, N. J., Hames, P., Brown, J. S., & Sivell, S. (2014). A randomized, placebo-controlled trial of online cognitive behavioral therapy for chronic insomnia disorder delivered via an automated media-rich web application. *Sleep*, 37(9), 1443–1453.

Frates, B., Bonnet, J., Joseph, R., & Peterson, J. (2020). *Lifestyle medicine handbook, an introduction to the power of healthy habits* (2nd ed.). Health Living.

Fredrickson, B. (2004). The broaden–and–build theory of positive emotions. *Phil. Trans. R. Soc. Lond. B3591367.* https://doi.org/10.1098/rstb.2004.1512

Fredrickson, B. L., & Losada, M. F. (2005). Positive affect and the complex dynamics of human flourishing. *Am Psychol.* 60(7), 678–686.

Gander, F., Proyer, R., Ruch, W., & Wyss, T. (2013). Strength-based positive interventions: Further evidence for their potential in enhancing well-being and alleviating depression. *Journal of Happiness Studies*, 14(4), 1241–1259. https://doi-org.elib.tcd.ie/10.1007/s10902-012-9380-0

Garrett, N., & Sharot, T. (2017). Optimistic update bias holds firm: Three tests of robustness following Shah et al. *Consciousness and Cognition: An International Journal*, 50, 12–22. https://doi.org/10.1016/j.concog.2016.10.013

Gong, H., Ni, C. X., Liu, Y. Z., Zhang, Y., Su, W. J., Lian, Y. J., Peng, W., & Jiang, C. L. (2016). Mindfulness meditation for insomnia: A meta-analysis of randomized controlled trials. *Journal of Psychosomatic Research*, 89, 1–6. https://doi.org/10.1016/j.jpsychores.2016.07.016

Gujar, N., McDonald, S. A., Nishida, M., & Walker, M. P. (2011). A role for REM sleep in recalibrating the sensitivity of the human brain to specific emotions. *Cerebral Cortex, 21*(1), 115–123. https://doi.org/10.1093/cercor/bhq064

Hamilton, N. A., Nelson, C. A., Stevens, N., & Kitzman, H. (2007). Sleep and psychological well-being. *Social Indicators Research, 82*(1), 147–163. https://doi.org/10.1007/s11205-006-9030-1

Hughes, N., & Burke, J. (2018). Sleeping with the frenemy: How restricting 'bedroom use' of smartphones impacts happiness and wellbeing. *Computers in Human Behavior, 85*, 236–244. https://doi.org/10.1016/j.chb.2018.03.047

Joseph, S. (2013). *What doesn't kill us: The new psychology of posttraumatic growth.* Basic Books.

King, L. A. & Miner, K. N. (2000). Writing about the benefits of traumatic events: Implications for physical health. *Pers Soc Psychol Bull.* 26(2). https://doi.org/10.1177/0146167200264008

Kluemper, D. H., Little, L. M., & DeGroot T. (2009). State or trait: Effects of state optimism on job-related outcomes. *J Org Behav.* 30(2), 209–231. https://doi.org/10.1002/job.591

Kredlow, M. A., Capozzoli, M. C., Hearon, B. A., Calkins, A. W., & Otto, M. W. (2015). The effects of physical activity on sleep: A meta-analytic review. *Journal of Behavioral Medicine, 38*(3), 427–449. https://doi.org/10.1007/s10865-015-9617-6

Látos, M., Lázár, G., Ondrik, Z., Szederkényi, E., Hódi, Z., Horváth, Z., & Csabai, M. (2022). Positive psychology intervention to improve recovery after renal transplantation: A randomized controlled trial. *Journal of Contemporary Psychotherapy: On the Cutting Edge of Modern Developments in Psychotherapy, 52*(1), 35–44. https://doi.org/10.1007/s10879-021-09515-6

Li, J.-B., Dou, K., & Liang, Y. (2021). The relationship between presence of meaning, search for meaning, and subjective well-being: A three-level meta-analysis based on the meaning in life questionnaire. *Journal of Happiness Studies, 22*(1), 467–489. https://doi.org/10.1007/s10902-020-00230-y

Lollies, F., Schnatschmidt, M., Bihlmeier, I., Genuneit, J., In-Albnon, T., Holtmann, M., Legenbauer, T., & Schlarb, A. A. (2022). Associations of sleep and emotion regulation processes in childhood and adolescence – A systematic review, report of methodological challenges and future directions. *Sleep Sci, 15*(4), 490–514. https://doi.org/10.5935/1984-0063.20220082.

Lopresti, A. L., Hood, S. D., & Drummond, P. D. (2013). A review of lifestyle factors that contribute to important pathways associated with major depression: Diet, sleep and exercise. *Journal of Affective Disorders, 148*(1), 12–27.

Michel, A., Groß, C., Hoppe, A., González, M. M. G., Steidle, A., & O'Shea, D. (2021). Mindfulness and positive activities at work: Intervention effects on motivation-related constructs, sleep quality, and fatigue. *Journal of Occupational & Organizational Psychology, 94*(2), 309–337. https://doi.org/10.1111/joop.12345

Moskowitz, J. T., & Saslow, L. R. (2014). Health and psychology: The importance of positive affect. In M. M. Tugade, M. N. Shiota, & L. D. Kirby (Eds.), *Handbook of positive emotions.* The Guilford Press.

Ng, M. Y., & Wong, W. S. (2012). The differential effects of gratitude and sleep on psychological distress in patients with chronic pain. *J Health Psychol, 18*(2). https://doi.org/10.1177/1359105312439733

O'Donovan, R., & Burke, J. (2022). Factors associated with post-traumatic growth in healthcare professionals: A systematic review of the literature. *Healthcare (Basel, Switzerland), 10*(12), 2524. https://doi.org/10.3390/healthcare10122524

Ong, A. D., Kim, S., Young, S., & Steptoe, A. (2017). Positive affect and sleep: A systematic review. *Sleep Med Rev, 35*, 21–32. https://doi.org/10.1016/j.smrv.2016.07.006

Ong, J. C., Manber, R., Segal, Z., Xia, Y., Shapiro, S., & Wyatt, J. K. (2012). A randomized controlled trial of mindfulness meditation for chronic insomnia. *Sleep, 35*(12), 1601–1608. https://doi.org/10.5665/sleep.4010.

Pérusse, A. D., De Koninck, J., Pedneault-Drolet, M., Ellis, J. G., & Bastien, C. H. (2016). REM dream activity of insomnia sufferers: A systematic comparison with good sleepers. *Sleep Medicine, 20*, 147–154. https://doi.org/10.1016/j.sleep.2015.08.007

Phelan, C. H., Love, G. D., Ryff, C. D., Brown, R. L., & Heidrich, S. M. (2010). Psychosocial predictors of changing sleep patterns in aging women: A multiple pathway approach. *Psychology and Aging, 25*(4), 858–866. https://doi.org/10.1037/a0019622

Roepke, A. M., Jayawickreme, E., & Riffle, O. M. (2014). Meaning and health: A systematic review. *Applied Research in Quality of Life, 9*(4), 1055–1079. https://doi.org/10.1007/s11482-013-9288-9

Ryff, C. D., Singer, B. H., & Dienberg Love, G. (2004). Positive health: connecting well-being with biology. *Philosophical Transactions of the Royal Society of London. Series B, Biological Sciences, 359*(1449), 1383–1394. https://doi.org/10.1098/rstb.2004.1521

Saksvik-Lehouillier, I., Saksvik, S. B., Dahlberg, J., Tanum, T. K., Ringen, H., Karlsen, H. R., Smedbol, T., Sorengard, T. A., Stople, M., Kallestad, H., & Olsen, A. (2020). Mild to moderate partial sleep deprivation is associated with increased impulsivity and decreased affect in young adults. *Sleep*, 1–10. https://doi.org/10.1093/sleep/zsaa078

Sarin, S., Motta, M., & Gobble, J. E. (2022). *The practitioner's guide to lifestyle medicine*. Healthy Learning.

Schippers, M. C. & Ziegler, N. (2019). Life crafting as a way to find purpose and meaning in life. *Front Psychol.* 10, 2778. https://doi.org/10.3389/fpsyg.2019.02778

Seligman, M. E. P. (2006). *Learned optimism: How to change your mind and your life*. Vintage.

Sharot, T. (2011). *The optimism bias: A tour of the irrationally positive brain*. Pantheon/Random House.

Sheikh-Wu, S. F., Anglade, D., Gattamorta, K., & Downs, C. A. (2023). Relationships between colorectal cancer Survivors' positive psychology, symptoms, and quality of life. *Clinical Nursing Research, 32*(1), 171–184. https://doi.org/10.1177/10547738221113385.

Smith, M. T., Perlis, M. L., Park, A., Smith, M. S., Pennington, J., Giles, D. E., & Buysse, D. J. (2002). Comparative meta-analysis of pharmacotherapy and behavior therapy for persistent insomnia. *American Journal of Psychiatry, 159*(1), 5–11. https://doi.org/10.1176/appi.ajp.159.1.5.

Steger, M. (2017). Meaning in life and wellbeing. In M. Slade, L. Oades, & A. Jarden (Eds.), *Wellbeing, recovery and mental health* (pp. 75–85). Routledge.

Steptoe, A., O'Donnell, K., Marmot, M., & Wardle, J. (2008). Positive affect, psychological well-being, and good sleep. *Journal of Psychosomatic Research, 64*(4), 409–415. https://doi.org/10.1016/j.jpsychores.2007.11.008.

Tedeschi, R. G., & Calhoun, L. G. (2004). Target article: Posttraumatic growth: Conceptual foundations and empirical evidence. *Psychological Inquiry, 15*(1), 1–18. https://doi.org/10.1207/s15327965pli1501_01.

Uchino, B., Cribbet, M., Grey, R., Cronan, S., Trettevik, R., & Smith, T. (2017). Dispositional optimism and sleep quality: A test of mediating pathways. *Journal of Behavioral Medicine, 40*(2), 360–365. https://doi.org/10.1007/s10865-016-9792-0.

Walker, M. P., & van der Helm, E. (2009). Overnight therapy? The role of sleep in emotional brain processing. *Psychological Bulletin, 135*(5), 731–748. https://doi.org/10.1037/a0016570.

Watson, N. F., Badr, M. S., Belenky, G., Bliwise, D. L., Buxton, O. M., Buysse, D., Dinges, D. F., Gangwisch, J., Grander, M. A., Kushisa, C., Malhotra, R. K., Martin, J. L., Patel, S. R., Quan, S. F., & Tasali, E. (2015). Recommended amount of sleep for A healthy adult: A joint consensus statement of the American academy of sleep medicine and sleep research society. *Sleep., 38*(6), 843–844. https://doi.org/10.5665/sleep.4716.

Weitzer, J., Papantoniou, K., Lázaro-Sebastià, C., Seidel, S., Klösch, G., & Schernhammer, E. (2021). The contribution of dispositional optimism to understanding insomnia symptomatology: Findings from a cross-sectional population study in Austria. *Journal of Sleep Research, 30*(1), e13132. https://doi.org/10.1111/jsr.13132.

Wood, A. M., Joseph, S., Lloyd, J., & Atkins, S. (2009). Gratitude influences sleep through the mechanism of pre-sleep cognitions. *J Psychosom Res, 66*(1), 43–48. https://doi.org/10.1016/j.jpsychores.2008.09.002.

Worley, S. L. (2018). The detrimental effects of inadequate sleep on health and public safety drive an explosion of sleep research. *Pharmacy and Therapeutics, 43*(12), 758–763.

Yoo, S. S., Gujar, N., Hu, P., Jolesz, F. A., & Walker, M. P. (2007). The human emotional brain without sleep—A prefrontal amygdala disconnect. *Curr Biol, 17*(20), 877–878. https://doi.org/10.1016/j.cub.2007.08.007.

6 The Role of Positive Psychology in Substance Use Harm Reduction and Recovery

Chapter Overview

This chapter provides highlights from the science that examines the role of positive psychology in substance use. We provide practical clinical applications, including coaching strategies, that leverage positive psychology to support avoidance of risky substance use, treat mild addictions, and achieve harm reduction from substance use. Interventions aligned with the PERMA model, appreciative inquiry, and character strengths are described. The role of reducing substance use in promoting mental and emotional, as well as physical wellbeing, in a clinical practice that emphasizes positive health is discussed.

Introduction

Substance use disorders represent a major public health issue, affecting millions of people worldwide. About 270 million people (or about 5.5% of the global population aged from 15 to 64) had psychoactive drugs in the previous year and an estimated 35 million are affected by substance use disorders. More than 42 million years of healthy life are lost due to substance use, according to the World Health Organization (WHO, Drugs. https://www.who.int/health-topics/drugs-psychoactive). Substance use disorders can lead to a range of negative outcomes, including physical and mental health problems and social isolation, as well as financial difficulties and legal issues.

Therefore, a comprehensive healthy lifestyle includes avoidance of risky substance use – tobacco, alcohol, illicit drugs, and misuse of prescription drugs – or reducing harm from substance use to prevent physical and mental consequences (Velten et al., 2014). Lifestyle medicine practitioners and health care teams can offer evidence-based brief interventions, such as motivational

DOI: 10.4324/9781003428909-6

interviewing, integrated with positive psychology approaches. However, these require further study as stand-alone treatments.

Theoretical Underpinnings of Positive Psychology Relevant to Substance Use

Substance use avoidance and recovery can be achieved and supported through positive psychology applications as part of the prevention and treatment plan. These interventions aim to promote positive emotions (such as gratitude, hope, and joy), enhance positive behaviors (such as seeking social support), and foster positive cognitions (such as optimism and self-efficacy) that serve as essential underpinnings for successful outcomes. Theoretical frameworks for this approach include the broaden-and-build theory of positive emotions, the self-determination theory of motivation, and the social cognitive theory of self-regulation.

The broaden-and-build theory of positive emotions posits that positive emotions broaden individuals' attentional focus and cognitive scope, allowing them to perceive a wider range of possibilities and resources. Positive emotions also build psychological and social resources over time, which can lead to improved wellbeing and resilience. The self-determination theory of motivation suggests that individuals have three innate psychological needs: autonomy, competence, and relatedness. When these needs are satisfied, individuals are more likely to engage in positive behaviors and experience positive emotions. The social cognitive theory of self-regulation posits that individuals can develop self-efficacy beliefs through observing and modeling the behavior of others, receiving feedback, and experiencing success in achieving goals (Bandura, 1991; Fredrickson, 2004; Ryan & Deci, 2000; Tougas et al, 2015).

Positive Psychology Strategies to Address Substance Use

Substance use behavior change can be facilitated using motivational interviewing (Miller & Rollnick, 2013), cognitive behavioral, and positive psychology techniques (McHugh et al., 2011). Reframing the use of alcohol or other drug use as a lifestyle behavior may free up the individual to view decreases in substance use as attainable. The positive psychology goal of a pleasant, engaged and meaningful life can empower this change. Paying attention to what is going well in one's life and pleasant experiences, practicing gratitude, positive reappraisal, leveraging character strengths, and increasing positive affect have been implemented in recovery from alcohol use, smoking, and other drug addictions (Krentzman, 2013).

A key construct in the role of positive psychology for addressing substance use is its capacity to fulfill basic psychological needs. Increasing positive experiences can help counter the motivation to turn to substance use and escape unpleasant, negative life experiences or memories of traumatic events. In fact, it has been posited that the lack of PERMA and related positive activities produces an imbalance in the brain reward centers that can lead to starting or increasing substance use (Stone, 2022). Positive psychology intervention (PPI) can restore that imbalance. For example, mindfulness meditation can increase activity in brain regions associated with emotion regulation and attention (Guendelman et al., 2017). Gratitude interventions have been shown to increase activity in the prefrontal cortex, a brain region associated with positive emotion processing and decision-making (Fox et al., 2015). Positive social support interventions have been linked to changes in brain activity in regions associated with social cognition and reward processing (Bhanji & Delgado, 2014). These kinds of brain changes can impact substance use behavior.

Such PPIs can be incorporated into systems of care. For example, eight weekly workshops based on principles of happiness, optimism, strengths, and gratitude were offered to adolescents attending an alcohol and drug treatment service with a rise in positive emotions and a decline in substance use. Although that pilot study was small and recommended a full-scale study, it did confirm the feasibility of positive psychology programs as part of substance misuse care (Akhtar & Boniwell, 2010).

However, many individuals do not seek therapy due to societal stigma and other barriers; hence positive psychology activities can be self-initiated. PPIs and positive health approaches in clinical settings and self-care assisted by online, digital, and community programs may offer an effective framework for substance use treatment and prevention strategies and have the potential to be culturally tailored for greater engagement (Crookes, 2018; Krentzman, 2013).

Empirical Evidence for PPIs in Substance Use Management

Empirical studies suggest that positive psychology approaches, including mindfulness, gratitude, and strengths-based practices, can strengthen other interventions to reduce substance use and promote successful substance use treatment.

Mindfulness-Based Interventions

As stress has a mediating role in substance-seeking behaviors (Sinha, 2008), not surprisingly, mindfulness-based treatments, such as stress reduction (MBSR) and mindfulness-based relapse prevention (MBRP), have been shown to be effective for individuals struggling with substance use. These treatments may reduce substance use and improve psychological wellbeing in individuals with substance use disorders through their impact on self-regulation (Garland & Howard, 2018; Katz & Toner, 2014; Korecki et al., 2020; Witkiewitz et al., 2005, 2013). MBSR is a group-based intervention that includes mindfulness meditation, gentle yoga, and body awareness exercises. MBRP is a relapse prevention program that integrates mindfulness practices with cognitive-behavioral techniques. Both interventions aim to help individuals develop a non-judgmental awareness of their thoughts, emotions, and physical sensations, and to cultivate acceptance, self-compassion, and emotional regulation skills (Katz & Toner, 2014; Korecki et al., 2020).

A randomized controlled trial (RCT) found that individuals with substance use disorders who received MBRP had a lower rate of relapse and longer abstinence periods compared to those who received standard relapse prevention treatment (Bowen et al, 2014). Also, mindfulness therapy in one RCT was found to be more effective than cognitive behavior therapy in an RCT for alcohol and/or cocaine use (Brewer et al., 2009). Another RCT found that individuals who received mindfulness therapy for smoking cessation showed a greater reduction in cigarette use during treatment and maintained this at 17-week follow-up compared to the group that received the American Lung Association freedom from smoking treatment (Brewer et al., 2011).

Several other studies show the relevance and potential efficacy of mindfulness-based interventions for substance use, including retention of women in residential treatment centers (Black, 2019). However, further study is needed to evaluate the outcomes of such interventions, especially in different groups, as race and ethnicity may interact with the results (Greenfield et al., 2018).

Gratitude Interventions

Gratitude interventions – activities that promote feelings of gratitude, such as writing gratitude letters or keeping a gratitude journal – have also been shown to reduce substance use and improve psychological wellbeing. A RCT of individuals with substance use disorders found that those who participated in a gratitude intervention improved their mental health outcomes, including increased gratitude, hope, and a sense of wellbeing, compared to those who received treatment as usual (Krentzman et al., 2015). However, gratitude has been associated with maintaining the status quo, hence, may be contraindicated, for high frequency drinkers (Krentzman, 2017). Aligning with this finding, individuals already in recovery benefited from gratitude journaling by reinforcing the positive aspects of recovery (Krentzman et al., 2023).

Strengths-Based Interventions

Certain character strengths have been associated with lower substance use. In a study of college students, higher temperance scores were associated with abstinence, lower-risk drinking, and fewer consequences among heavy drinkers. Justice and transcendence were independently associated with abstinence-only (Logan et al., 2010). Hence, strengths-based assessment and interventions that aim to identify and cultivate the use of individual strengths, such as creativity and optimism, and enhance psychological wellbeing may serve as helpful tools to reduce substance use in individuals with substance use disorders (Ezell et al., 2023).

A review of the literature suggests that a strengths-based approach in populations with substance use disorders can serve as an effective adjunct or alternative to traditional treatment (Berg, 2016). Specific character strengths that have emerged in the studies that may be salient to substance use recovery are wisdom, integrity, vitality, humility, forgiveness, kindness, love, hope, and spirituality (Selvam, 2015).

To date, the addiction (sexual, alcoholic etc.) research is focused mainly on developing a limited number of character strengths (Burke & Stephens, 2018). They usually are the strengths of spirituality and gratitude (Zemansky, 2006). However, considering that strengths are unique expressions of each human being and they all should be used to help us live a good life, more effort is required to incorporate all of the ones that are relevant for each individual to help patients with addiction.

When character strengths were included in a therapeutic approach to smoking cessation, they showed a significant reduction in addictive behavior (Day et al., 2014). Both clients and therapists also reported how enjoyable sessions were when they discussed strengths, instead of clients' deficits and how they can be used to help them accomplish their addiction goals. A similar approach can be applied in any discussions between physicians and their patients, whereby physicians could ask questions about what strengths their patients have, how they have used those strengths in the past, and how they can use them again to instigate lasting change.

Furthermore, past research indicates that a brief reflection on a patients' strengths, prior to seeing the patient, significantly improves the provider-patient relationship and therapeutic outcomes (Flückiger & Grosse, 2008). Therefore, exploring patients' strengths and drawing upon them can prove useful to physicians and the health team.

Activities that Promote Positive Affect and Their Role in Substance Use

Positive emotions are a protective factor for enhancing abstinence-related action tendencies in individuals who are dependent on methamphetamine (Carrico et al., 2013). Experiencing higher levels of positive emotions was associated with a stronger belief that they can manage their methamphetamine triggers. Most importantly, however, this study also showed that those who experienced higher levels of positive emotions during a 30-day study involving urine sample testing for toxicology screening were using less substance in this period. Similarly, a study with alcohol-dependent out-patients showed that positive affect was directly associated with lower craving levels (McHugh et al., 2013). Furthermore, positive affect significantly reduces relapse in drug addicts (Zand et al., 2017). Thus, evidence suggests that positive affect plays a significant role in reducing substance abuse.

A study with over 500 adults who described themselves as recovering from substance abuse participated in an online wellbeing program (Hoeppner et al., 2019b). Participants incorporated one short (approximately four-minute) wellbeing activity in their daily routine. The most effective activity in this program was "Reliving Happy Moments," followed by "Savoring," and "Rose, Thorn, and Bud," described in the box. Interestingly, the gratitude activity (think back to three good things that happened to you in the last 24 hours) and the kindness activity (performing or witnessing acts of kindness) were the least effective of all the wellbeing exercises.

Reliving Happy Moments (Adapted from Hoeppner et al., 2019b)

Each day, browse through the pictures you have saved on your smartphone, computer, or lying around. Select one that brings back a happy memory. Relive the happy moment.

Savoring (Adapted from Hoeppner et al., 2019b)

Think about a positive experience you have actively savored in the last 24 hours. Consider what made the experience positive and think about what made you appreciate it at the time. These experiences could include everyday moments worthwhile savoring, such as enjoying tea. If you have not experienced any active savoring moments in the last 24 hours, reflect on the positive experience you are likely to have in the next 24 hours that you can savor.

Rose, Thorn, and Bud (Adapted from Hoeppner et al., 2019b)

What is the BEST thing that you have experienced in the last 24 hours (your rose), the WORST thing you have experienced in the last 24 hours (your thorn), and the thing you are most looking forward to in the next 24 hours (your bud)?

Balanced Time Perspectives

What is interesting about the activities in the previous section is that they draw on various time perspectives, especially encouraging participants to create positive emotions from past experiences. This approach of crowding out negative memories by bringing positive past events into consciousness has been used extensively in time perspective therapy with war veterans (Zimbardo et al., 2012). What matters is that individuals have a balanced time perspective that allows them to draw effectively from their psychological resources. Any form of imbalance may result in pathologies or unwanted behaviors. For example, a study with gamblers found that they had a strongly developed present hedonic time perspective and a less developed future time perspective (Hodgins & Engel, 2002), meaning that they were not able to tap into the future to identify the consequences of their behavior in the present, which may have resulted in taking their gambling to an unsustainable level.

Substance misuse has a slightly different time perspective pattern, whereby individuals who did not spend much time in the future reported higher levels of substance abuse; however, the results were inconsistent (Keough et al., 1999). A far better predictor of substance abuse was spending significantly more time in the present. Even after controlling for individuals' personality differences, a present-time perspective (hedonic or fatalistic) was associated with more frequent substance abuse. For example, those spending time predominantly in the here and now were more likely to drink more alcohol on a single occasion, more over a weekend, and consumed more alcohol in the past month compared to those whose present-time perspective was less prominent.

Humor

A sense of humor is rarely considered an important characteristic associated with substance abuse. Nevertheless, an extensive research sample indicates that individuals who have experienced alcohol abuse problems tend to display the least effective humor type, i.e. aggressive (Schermer et al., 2023). According to the humor style theory, there are four different styles: (1) affiliative humor, (2) self-enhancing humor, (3) aggressive humor, and (4) self-defeating humor (Martin, 2007). The first two types of humor are adaptive in that affiliative humor is a light-hearted type that brings people together, e.g. a joke about current affairs that everyone understands. Self-enhancing humor aims to improve our mood by reflecting on a funny situation we find ourselves in, e.g. reframing a problematic situation in a light-hearted way. Affiliative and self-enhancing types of humor serve us well as they intend to make light of challenging life without harming others. The two maladaptive humor types are self-defeating humor based on self-deprecation, e.g. ridiculing self.

This type of humor is perceived by some researchers as semi-adaptive, depending on circumstances. If a person believes in the negative things they say about themselves and it impacts them negatively (e.g. "I am such a klutz"), it is maladaptive. However, self-deprecation can also bring people closer together when, for example, in a meeting, a person in authority uses self-deprecation; they may be perceived as more humane. There are, however, no instances when the aggressive type of humor is adaptive. It is about belittling an individual or groups of people, e.g. jokes about minority groups. This type of humor manipulates others and threatens them with ridicule. This is the type of humor associated with higher levels of substance abuse. The box offers suggestions for activities that can be used with individuals abusing substances to help them develop the self-enhancing type of humor.

Three Funny Things (Adapted from Gander et al., 2013)

Every evening, before going to bed, set aside 15 minutes and write down the three funniest things that happened to you that day. Reflect on the reasons why they happened.

Solving a Stressful Situation Humorously (Adapted from Wellenzohn et al., 2016)

Whenever you experience a stressful situation, reflect on ways in which you could have resolved it in a funny way.

Applying Humor (Adapted from Wellenzohn et al., 2016)

At the end of the day, reflect on all the humorous situations that happened to you that day. Consider how you can build more humor into the next day by adding activities and situations that make you laugh using adaptive types of humor.

Applications of Positive Psychology to Manage Substance Use

Just as with the other lifestyle pillars, a health practitioner can apply a variety of positive psychology techniques to help patients reduce risky substance use. These techniques can also assist management and treatment of mild substance use disorders.

The PERMA framework, appreciative inquiry and the five A's can be adapted to assist patients with decreasing substance use or minimizing substance use harm. Also, positive psychology activities, such as gratitude practice, mindfulness meditation, improved coping skills and strengthened social support, may be applied to buffer against adversities and bolster mental health to help avoid risky substance use. The list below outlines how the PERMA framework can be used to address substance use.

Application of PERMA in the Context of Substance Use

P—Positive emotions: Savor positive feelings and experiences in your life, instead of turning to substance use.
- What kinds of activities bring forth positive feelings and a sense of vitality and energy? How can you incorporate these into your life, as you decrease your substance use?
- How can you pay attention to and savor positive/happy experiences when you feel the urge for your substance of choice?

E—Engagement (Flow): Notice how you can enhance joy by doing positive activities in which you get fully immersed, for example when creating something artistic, playing music, dancing, and gardening.
- What activities have you done in the past or recently that give you a sense of flow?
- What new activities that could produce a sense of flow would you like to try?
- How can you increase or add such activities, as you decrease your substance use?

R—Relationships: Identify how you can increase positive social interactions.
- What relationships are important to you and how can you spend more time with those individuals in healthy ways without substance use?
- What people can support you in your goal of decreasing or eliminating your substance use?

M—Meaning: Pay attention to how reducing or eliminating substance use aligns with your values and what is meaningful to you.
- What are meaningful ways you can engage with your family and friends in place of substance use?
- What activities can you increase or add that align with your life purpose and feel meaningful?

A—Achievement: Reflect on recent and past accomplishments. Notice and celebrate any progress toward your goal of decreasing your substance use and improving your life.
- What activities give you a genuine sense of accomplishment? How can you increase these, as you decrease your substance use?

- What small steps have you achieved toward your substance use reduction or elimination goal? For example, having self-compassion about your substance use situation and bravery to speak about it openly and seek help

The Five A's Emphasizing Positive Psychology

The five A's model of ask, advise, assess, and assist has often been used as a practical guide for the steps to manage behavior change. The traditional steps can be modified to include or emphasize positive psychology constructs.

Ask: Ask the individual when they have been using substances most responsibly or avoiding use? Under what circumstances? With whom and when? What positive feelings did they have during these circumstances?

Advise: State the recommendation to eliminate or decrease the substance. Discuss how they can recreate the circumstances when they were able to avoid substances – with a focus on gaining the associated positive feelings, such as a sense of pride and achievement.

Assess: Check the individual's readiness to make a change in their substance use habits and consider the positive aspects of making the change.

Assist: Conduct motivation interviewing with an emphasis on envisioning a positive future in which they reach and sustain their goal – with the expected benefits. Inquire about who can support them and how can they reward themselves for progress – even small progress – in healthy ways. Help them develop an action plan.

Arrange: Discuss next steps and include a plan to evaluate what goes well with each step toward achieving the action plan.

Appreciative Inquiry to Support a Decrease Substance Use

The health care provider and team can use appreciative inquiry to help build a positive process that can advance taking action toward substance use harm reduction and avoiding risky use. The process can promote self-compassion, use of strengths, and positive emotions that bring attention away from urges to use substances.

Discovery: What is good now?
- What kinds of habits do you have now that support your health and happiness?
- How do you work on limiting your substance use?
- What positive activities do you do now that help distract you from substance use?
- What strengths do you use now to help manage your substance use?

Dream: What changes are possible that would create joy and reduce the desire or need for substance use?
- What are possible healthy activities that bring joy and hope?
- In what ways would it be possible to increase or add such activities, and divert from the urge for substance use?

Design: What positive changes could you make in your life?
- What favorite positive activities could you add to your life or increase, while you decrease or eliminate your substance use?
- With whom could you connect to support your goal to avoid risky substance use?
- What strengths could you use to achieve and maintain your goal to decrease risky substance use?

Destiny: What positive changes are you confident you can make?
- What action plan are you confident you can do to increase activities that are a source of joy, pride, or other positive feelings while decreasing your substance use?
- Which strengths will you use to achieve your substance use action plan?
- What are healthy ways you can reward yourself for achieving your action plan?

Positive Health Integrated into Lifestyle Medicine Core Competencies: Treating Substance Use Disorder

As we've seen, PPIs can be integrated into substance use avoidance, reduction, or treatment plans as part of a comprehensive healthy lifestyle plan, or as a component of standard counseling programs, such as motivational interviewing (Miller & Rollnick, 2013), that help patients move through the stages of the behavior change transtheoretical model (Prochaska et al., 1992). Lifestyle medicine competencies provide guidance for this clinical work. Several lifestyle medicine (LM) competencies for substance use treatment can be grounded in positive psychology and positive health strategies and principles.

- When describing the health effects of tobacco, alcohol, and other frequently used substances and the benefits of cessation, highlight the impact of substance use cessation or reduction on emotional and mental health improvements and the capacity to achieve the envisioned positive future and goals.
- When creating patient-centered substance use treatment plans according to practice guidelines and harnessing behavioral interventions, include positive activities to increase positive emotions that drive substance-use avoidance or reduction.

Table 6.1 Expanded positive health competencies: Treating substance use disorder

Lifestyle medicine competencies	Positive health expansion
Describe the health effects of tobacco, alcohol, and other frequently used substances and the benefits of cessation	Describe the impact of substance use cessation or reduction on emotional and mental health improvements, and on the capacity to achieve one's envisioned positive future goals
Create patient-centered substance use treatment plans using practice guidelines and behavioral interventions	Create substance-use treatment plans with positive activities to increase positive emotions that drive the behavior changes, i.e. the link between increased vitality, hope, and capacity to achieve and sustain substance-use avoidance or reduction
Integrate behavior therapy with pharmacotherapy for tobacco and other substance use disorder plans, and refer to a substance use disorder specialist when indicated	Emphasize positive psychology approaches, including appreciative inquiry, for highlighting the positive aspects of avoiding or reducing substance use; describe how success with substance use reduction amplifies positive health

- When integrating behavior therapy with pharmacotherapy for tobacco and other substance use disorder plans, emphasize positive psychology approaches, including appreciative inquiry for highlighting positive aspects of avoiding or reducing substance use on the road to positive health.

Table 6.1 lists the competencies for treating substance use disorder in the left column and provides suggestions in the right column for a positive health expansion for each competency.

Perspectives on Practicing from the Inside Out – Substance Use

When helping patients address their substance use, we need to have an awareness of our own experiences and biases about substance use. Each of us has a comfort zone for substance use from not tolerating it at all to feeling that some use is acceptable. Of course, that comfort level will vary based on whether the substance is tobacco, alcohol, illicit substances, or use of prescription medications not as prescribed.

Self-awareness of our attitudes and reframing of our mindset to be open and to nonjudgmentally connect with our patients about their substance use can help us approach this health pillar from a place more effectively. A deep understanding is needed to make authentic connections about any behavior change; it is particularly essential for the substance use pillar. Patients may have an ear toward being judged and, if they sense they are being judged, they may shut down the authentic discussion needed to develop steps in the behavior change and healing process.

As providers, we also need to help our patients avert the stigma of substance use by society. PPIs can help counteract the negative stereotypes and stigmatization that individuals face when using substances, especially individuals with substance use disorders. By highlighting individuals' strengths and positive attributes, we can help reduce shame and self-blame and promote a more positive and hopeful outlook on recovery.

Spotlight on Smoking Cessation with Positive Psychology Approaches

As smoking cessation is a common substance use issue addressed in health care practice, we'd like to highlight the role of positive psychology for tobacco use management. In addition to well-known coaching techniques, such as motivational interviewing (Miller & Rollnick, 2013) and cognitive behavioral therapy (Killen et al., 2008; Lightfoot et al., 2020; Vinci, 2020), positive psychology techniques, may be considered, especially when combined with the former to address mood issues (USHHS, 2020). Positive psychology approaches may help counter negative effects, such as anxiety, that can trigger smoking urges; they can work through self-regulatory and self-efficacy processes to support an individual to achieve goals to limit or stop smoking (Vidrine et al., 2016). These techniques can be applied in traditional clinical settings and via phone and app-based programs (Hoeppner et al., 2019a).

Moreover, specific positive emotions have been correlated with lower likelihood of next-day relapse during quitting attempts: high levels of happiness and relaxation and increasing levels of these emotions and enthusiasm (Vinci et al., 2017).

A recent Cochrane Database review did not find a clear benefit of mindfulness-based smoking cessation interventions. However, the authors pointed out that variations in the type of interventions and quality of studies gave them low confidence in the available evidence (Jackson et al., 2022). More consistent studies are needed, including ones to determine the role of addressing mental and emotional health issues in smoking cessation.

In the meantime, practitioners may consider positive psychology approaches for patients undergoing smoking cessation treatment as additional support, not only when facing mental and emotional health issues, but also to boost positive emotions through multiple quit attempts often required for success. These approaches mirror previously listed interventions for substance use in general and are framed here as instructional messages:

Develop a Positive Mindset: Focusing on the positive aspects of quitting rather than the negative aspects of smoking has been a key technique for health coaches who offer smoking cessation counseling. Examples of what will be gained by quitting can include improved breathing to be active with one's grandchildren, better relationships with family members and friends who do not smoke, and increased pride and self-confidence for a major life and health achievement.

Cultivate Mindfulness: Being present at the moment and mindful of smoking triggers and then applying strategies for dealing with the triggers can be powerful. For example, if stress triggers the desire to smoke, MBSR techniques could help the individual cope without resorting to smoking.

Build Social Support: Social support is an important factor in quitting smoking. Building positive relationships and social support networks can be applied to quitting smoking by seeking out friends and family members who will encourage, motivate, and keep the individual accountable for reaching their desired goal of quitting smoking.

Focus on Positive Emotions: Joy, hope, pride, happiness, and gratitude can be leveraged in the process of quitting smoking. By focusing on the positive emotional experiences when making progress, those emotions can drive the nonconscious desire to do that behavior again. Every time one resists the urge to smoke, savoring the positive emotions of pride, accomplishment, and satisfaction can lead to that cycle of upward spiral of healthy lifestyle change.

Identify and Use Strengths: Smokers can identify their character strengths to help them quit smoking. Two examples include harnessing the strength of self-regulation to refrain from smoking and perseverance to try again after an unsuccessful quit attempt.

Case Study of Positive Health Approaches for Substance Use Management

Patient Background: John, a divorced, white, 45-year-old male computer engineer, presents with a history of high blood pressure and obesity. Medical records indicate he has struggled with a mild alcohol use disorder for several years. His drinking increased a year ago, and he entered a short inpatient treatment program. During the in-depth medical history review, he confessed that after discharge he increased his alcohol intake again. Although he was aiming to limit his beer drinking to a couple of beers on weekends, he admitted he often drank more than that. Recently this habit led to a major argument with his new girlfriend who threatened to leave unless he controlled his irritability and anger outbursts while drinking.

Assessment and Developing Treatment Plan: The provider discusses treatment options including PPIs. John is interested in making a change and motivated to avoid a relationship break-up. The provider explains that reducing his drinking could also help his blood pressure and improve his mood to help energize him and tackle other areas of his life, such as his weight. He is reluctant to try positive psychology approaches, as he feels that his problems are too deep-seated for such approaches to make a difference. He feels cutting out alcohol altogether is not realistic for him. The initial action plan he agrees to make is to decrease the number of drinks at one sitting to no more than two and to notify the health coach when he needs support.

Progress Update: John has difficulty sticking with the action plan. After his girlfriend breaks up with him, he reverts to his old habits of drinking on some weekdays, as well as weekends. A reprimand from his boss about letting deadlines slip and his loneliness drives John to return to the practice for further help. He is not willing to enter a treatment program again at this time.

Follow-up Visit: The health coach helps John develop a new action plan to eliminate drinking on weeknights and have no more than one drink a day on weekends. He is willing to try some other support to help him stay on track this time. The coach introduces him to gratitude journaling, taking a few minutes two times a week to write down three things for which he was grateful. In addition, the coach recommends John identify his character strengths and apply those in his plan to decrease his drinking. However, John is not interested. Lastly, the coach suggests a simple daily mindfulness practice, which John says he will consider.

Further Follow-Up – Gratitude Practice: In a follow-up call with the coach, John admits that he is having difficulty journaling about positive things, because he is consumed with negative emotions about himself and his life. The coach encourages him to embrace self-compassion – being as kind to himself as he might be to a friend who is struggling with a challenge; then write self-supportive thoughts along with the three good things. John finds he is able to sit and write positive reflections about the week on most Sundays; he gradually begins to notice small things that he appreciates in his life, such as a beautiful sunset or a kind word from a friend. As he continues the practice, he is naturally more able to notice the positive aspects of his life.

Further Follow-Up – Mindfulness Practice: John also reports that initially, he found it difficult to quiet his mind and focus on his breath. After a couple of attempts, he quit trying this mindfulness practice. On the bright side, after a few weeks of gratitude practice, which has lifted John's mood, he is open to trying mindfulness again. Over time, he feels more comfortable turning to mindfulness to manage his cravings for alcohol. By bringing his attention to the present moment, he is able to observe his thoughts and emotions without becoming overwhelmed by them.

Further Follow-up – Positive Self-Talk: With examples from the coach, John is also able to engage in positive self-talk during his cravings. He has learned to reframe negative thoughts in a more positive light. For example, when he found himself thinking "I'm never going to beat this addiction," he reframed the thought as "I'm taking steps every day to improve my life and overcome this addiction." By reframing his thoughts in this way, John is able to feel in control of his habits overall. The techniques of self-compassion and positive self-talk help buffer him from negative emotions in the face of setbacks that trigger the desire to drink alcohol. By applying these techniques, he finds it easier not to have any alcoholic drinks.

Outcome: John found that these interventions helped him to cultivate a more positive mindset and supported the self-efficacy he needed to maintain his sobriety over the long term.

Over time, John found that his outlook on life began to shift. He started to see himself as a person with strengths and positive qualities, rather than simply as an addict. He also found that his relationships with others improved, as he was better able to communicate his needs and emotions in a positive and constructive way.

Key Take-Aways: PPIs such as gratitude journaling, mindfulness meditation, use of character strengths, and positive self-talk can serve as powerful components of action plan to decrease risky substance use, or to treat mild substance use disorders. By buffering against negative emotions, bolstering self-efficacy and resiliency, and building resources to positively face the challenges of substance use recovery, PPIs serve as essential clinical and self-care tools.

Conclusion

Substance use disorders are a significant public health concern that requires effective treatment and prevention strategies. Studies suggest that PPIs can add value to traditional approaches for preventing problematic substance use and enhancing treatment.

Empirical evidence for PPIs, such as gratitude practice, meaningful activities aligned with a life purpose, and strengths-based interventions, points to their efficacy in improving psychological wellbeing. Although more high-quality research is needed, wellbeing that can result from these interventions may lead to reduced substance use and enhanced treatment outcomes in individuals with substance use disorders. Individuals struggling with substance misuse or addiction often experience feelings of hopelessness and despair. By introducing these patients to PPIs, practitioners can help patients break the cycle of negativity and cultivate empowering positive mindsets and emotions. In lifestyle medicine-oriented practices, PPIs can be harnessed into a comprehensive lifestyle program of the major pillars of a healthy lifestyle, which includes the avoidance of risky substance use or harm reduction from misuse. However, the limitations need to be considered. Some individuals may have underlying mental health issues or other challenges that require more intensive or specialized addiction treatment and should be referred out for this specialty care.

Future translational research should continue to explore the effectiveness of PPIs and the overarching positive health approach for substance use recovery and identify ways to optimize their implementation and delivery in clinical settings. In addition, more research is needed to fully understand the mechanisms through which PPIs may impact substance use. Another area of research that can assist practitioners is how to individualize PPIs for greater acceptability and better substance use outcomes in different age groups, cultures, and backgrounds, including a history of sexual abuse or other trauma.

Despite these limitations, practitioners can leverage some promising research results of positive psychology approaches in substance use counseling, treatment and self-care as part of the positive health approach. By focusing on promoting positive emotions, building strengths, and fostering positive relationships, individuals may be better equipped to prevent risky substance use, overcome substance use disorders, and maintain long-term recovery.

References

Akhtar, M., & Boniwell, I. (2010). Applying positive psychology to alcohol-misusing adolescents: A group intervention. *Groupwork, 20*(3), 6–31. https://doi.org/10.1921/095182410X576831

Bandura, A. (1991). Social cognitive theory of self-regulation. *Org Behav Hum Deci Proc, 50*(2), 248–287. https://doi.org/10.1016/0749-5978(91)90022-L

Berg, J. A. (2016). *Strengths-based treatment of substance use disorders: A critical analysis of the literature*. Pepperdine University ProQuest. Dissertations Publishing.

Bhanji, J. P., & Delgado, M. R. (2014). The social brain and reward: Social information processing in the human striatum. *Wiley Interdisc Rev Cogn Sci, 5*(1), 61–73. https://doi.org/10.1002/wcs.1266

Bowen, S., Witkiewitz, K., Clifasefi, S. L., Grow, S. L., Chawla, N., Hsu, S. H., Carroll, H. A., Harrop, E., Collins, S. E., Lustyk, M. K., & Larimer, M. E. (2014). Relative efficacy of mindfulness-based relapse prevention, standard relapse prevention, and treatment as usual for substance use disorders. *JAMA Psychiatry, 71*(5), 547–556. https://doi.org/10.1001/jamapsychiatry.2013.4546

Brewer, J. A., Sinha, R., Chen, J. A., Michalse, R. N., Babuscio, T. A., Nich, C., Grier, A., Bergquist, K. L., Reis, D. L., Potenza, M.N., Carroll, K.M., Rounsaville, B.J. (2009). Mindfulness training for smoking cessation: Results from a randomized controlled trial. *Drug Alcohol Dependence*, *119*(1–2), 72–80. https://doi.org/10.1016/j.drugalcdep.2011.05.027

Brewer, J. A., Sinha, R., Chen, J., Michalsen, A., Babuscio, R. N., Nich, T. A., Grier, C., Bergquist, A., Reis, K. L., Potenza, D. L., Carrol, M. N., & Rounsaville, K. M., B. J. (2009). Mindfulness training and stress reactivity in substance abuse: Results from a randomized, controlled stage I pilot study. *Subst. Abus.*, *30*(4), 306–317. https://doi.org/10.1080/08897070903250241

Burke, J., & Stephens, E. (2018). Applying positive psychology to sex addiction. In: T. Birchard, J. Benfield (Eds.), *The Routledge international handbook of sexual addiction* (pp. 235–246). Routledge/Taylor & Francis Group. https://doi.org/10.4324/9781315639512-21

Carrico, A. W., Woods, W. J., Siever, M. D., Discepola, M. V., Dilworth, S. E., Neilands, T. B., Miller, N., & Moskowitz, J. T. (2013). Positive affect and processes of recovery among treatment-seeking methamphetamine users. *Drug and Alcohol Dependence*, *132*(3), 624–629. https://doi.org/10.1016/j.drugalcdep.2013.04.018

Crookes, A. E. (2018). Positive psychology and the field of addiction – A proposal for a culturally relevant framework. *Middle East Journal of Positive Psychology*, *4*(1), 29–49.

Day, A. M., Clerkin, E. M., Spillane, N. S., & Kahler, C. W. (2014). Adapting positive psychology for smoking cessation. In A. C. Parks & S. M. Schueller (Eds.), *The Wiley Blackwell handbook of positive psychological interventions* (pp. 358–370). Wiley Blackwell. https://doi.org/10.1002/9781118315927.ch20

Ezell, J., Pho, M., Jaiswal, J., Ajayl, B. P., Gosnell, N., Kay, E. S., Eaton, E., & Bluthenthal, R. N. (2023). A systematic literature review of strength-based approaches to drug use management and treatment. *Clinical Social Work Journal*, *51*, 294–305. https://doi.org/10.1007/s10615-023-00874-2

Flückiger, C., & Grosse, H. M. (2008). Focusing the therapist's attention on the patient's strengths: A preliminary study to foster A mechanism of change in outpatient psychotherapy. *Journal of Clinical Psychology*, *64*(7), 876–890. https://doi.org/10.1002/jclp.20493

Fox, G. R., Kaplan, J., Damasio, H., & Damasio, A. (2015). Neural correlates of gratitude. *Front Psychol.*, *6*, 1491. https://doi.org/10.3389/fpsyg.2015.01491

Fredrickson, B. L. (2004). The broaden-and-build theory of positive emotions. *Phil Trans R Soc Lond.*, *359*, 1367–1377. https://doi.org/10.1098/rstb.2004.1512

Gander, F., Proyer, R. T., Ruch, W., & Wyss, T. (2013). Strength-based positive interventions: Further evidence for their potential in enhancing well-being and alleviating depression. *Journal of Happiness Studies: An Interdisciplinary Forum on Subjective Well-Being*, *14*(4), 1241–1259. https://doi.org/10.1007/s10902-012-9380-0

Garland, E. L., & Howard, M. O. (2018). Mindfulness-based treatment of addiction: Current state of the field and envisioning the next wave of research. *Addiction Science & Clinical Practice*, *13*(1), 14. https://doi.org/10.1037/ccp0000390

Greenfield, R. L., Roos, C., & Hagler, K. L., Stein, E., Bowen, S., & Witkiewitz (2018). Race/ethnicity and racial group composition moderate the effectiveness of mindfulness-based relapse prevention for substance use. *Addictive Behaviors*, *81*, 96–103.

Guendelman, S., Medeiros, S., & Rampes, H. (2017). Mindfulness and emotion regulation: Insights from neurobiological, psychological, psychological, and clinical studies. *Front Psychol*, *8*. https://doi.org/10.3389/fpsyg.2017.00220

Hodgins, D. C., & Engel, A. (2002). Future time perspective in pathological gamblers. *Journal of Nervous and Mental Disease, 190*(11), 775–780. https://doi.org/10.1097/00005053-200211000-00008

Hoeppner, B. B., Hoeppner, S. S., Carlon, H. A., Perez, G. K., Helmuth, E., Kahler, C. W., & Kelly, J. F. (2019a). Leveraging positive psychology to support smoking cessation in nondaily smokers using a smartphone app: Feasibilty and acceptability study. *JMIR Mhealth Uhealth, 7*(7), e13436. https://doi.org/10.2196/13436

Hoeppner, B. B., Schick, M. R., Carlon, H., & Hoeppner, S. S. (2019b). Do self-administered positive psychology exercises work in persons in recovery from problematic substance use? An online randomized survey. *Journal of Substance Abuse Treatment, 99*, 16–23. https://doi.org/10.1016/j.jsat.2019.01.006

Jackson, S., Brown, J., Norris, E., Livingstone-Banks, J., Hayes, E., & Lindson, N. (2022). Mindfulness for smoking cessation. *Cochrane Datbase Syst Rev, 4*, CD013696. https://doi.org/10.1002/14651858.CD013696

Katz, D., & Toner, B. (2014). A systematic review of sender differences in the effectiveness of mindfulness-based treatments for substance use disorders. *Mindfulness, 4*, 318–331. https://doi.org/10.1007/s12671-012-0132-3

Keough, K. A., Zimbardo, P. G., & Boyd, J. N. (1999). Who's smoking, drinking, and using drugs? Time perspective as a predictor of substance use. *Basic & Applied Social Psychology*, https://doi.org/10.1207/15324839951036498

Killen, J. D., Fortmann, S. P., & Schatzberg, A. F., Arredondo, C., Murphy G., Hayward, C., Celio, M., Cromp, D., Fong, D., & Pandurangi, M., (2008). Extended cognitive behavior therapy for cigarette smoking cessation. *Addiction, 103*(8), 1381–1390. https://doi.org/10.1111/j.1360-0443.2008.02273.x

Korecki, J. R., Schwebel, F. J., Votaw, V. R., & Witkiewitz, K. (2020). Mindfulness-based programs for substance use disorders: A systemic review of manualized treatments. *Substance Abuse Treatment, Prevention, and Policy, 2020*, 51. https://doi.org/10.1186/s13011-020-00293-3

Krentzman, A. R. (2013). Review of the application of positive psychology to substance use, addiction, and recovery research. *Psychology of Addictive Behaviors, 27*(1), 151–165. https://doi.org/10.1037/a0029897

Krentzman, A.R., Mannella, K. A., Hassett, A. K., Barnett, N. P., Higgins, M.M., & Meyer, P. S. (2015). Feasibility, Acceptability, and Impact of a web-based gratitude exercise among individuals in outpatient treatment for alcohol use disorder. *Journal of Positive Psychology.* 10(6), 477–488. https://doi.org/10.1080/17439760.2015.1015158

Krentzman, A. R. (2017). Gratitude, abstinence, and alcohol use disorders Report of a preliminary finding. *Journal of Substance Abuse Treatment.* 78:30–36. https://doi.org/10.1016/j.jsat.2017.04.013.

Krentzman, A. R., Hoeppner, B. B., Hoeppner, S. S., & Barnett, N. P. (2023). Development, feasibility, acceptability and impact of a positive psychology journaling intervention to support addiction recovery. *The Journal of Positive Psychology.* 18(4), 573–591. https://doi.org/10.1080/17439760.2022.2070531

Lightfoot, K., Panagiotaki, G., & Nobles, G. (2020). Effectiveness of psychological interventions for smoking cessation in adults with mental health problems: A systemic review. *Brit J Health Psychol, 25*(3), 615–638. https://doi.org/10.1111/bjhp.12431

Logan, D. E., Kilmer, J. R., & Mariatt, A. (2010). The virtuous drinker: Character virtues as correlates and moderators of college student drinking and consequences. *J Am College Health, 58*(4), 317–324. https://doi.org/10.1080/07448480903380326

Martin, R. A. (2007). *The psychology of humor: An integrative approach*. Elsevier.

McHugh, R. K., Hearon, B. A., & Otto, M. W. (2011). Cognitive-behavioral therapy for substance use disorders. *Psychiatr Clin North Am, 33*(3), 511–525. https://doi.org/10.1016/j.psc.2010.04.012

McHugh, R. K., Kaufman, J. S., Frost, K. H., Fitzmaurice, G. M., & Weiss, R. D. (2013). Positive affect and stress reactivity in alcohol-dependent outpatients. *Journal of Studies on Alcohol and Drugs, 74*(1), 152–157. https://doi.org/10.15288/jsad.2013.74.152

Miller, W. R., & Rollnick, S. (2013). *Motivational interviewing: Helping people change*. Guilford Press.

Park, C. L., Cho, D., & Kim, Y. (2015). Strengths-based interventions for individuals with alcohol use disorders: A qualitative study. *Journal of Substance Abuse Treatment, 53*, 1–8.

Prochaska, J. O., DiClemente, C. C., & Norcross, J. C. (1992). In search of how people change: Applications to addictive behaviors. *American Psychologist, 47*(9), 1102–1114. https://doi.org/10.1037/0003-066x.47.9.1102

Ryan, R., & Deci, E. L. (2000). Self-determination theory and the facilitation of intrinsic motivation, social development, and wellbeing. *American Psychologist, 55*(1), 68–78. https://doi.org/10.1037/0003-066X.55.1.68

Schermer, J. A., Kfrerer, L., & Lynskey, M. T. (2023). Alcohol dependence and humor styles. *Current Psychology, 42*(19), 16282–16286. https://doi.org/10.1007/s12144-019-00508-2

Selvam, S. G. (2015). Positive psychology's character strengths in addiction-spirituality research: A qualitative systemic literature review. *The Qualitative Report, 20*(4), 376–405. https://doi.org/10.46743/2160-3715/2015.2116

Sinha, R. (2008). Chronic stress, drug use, and vulnerability to addiction. *Annals of the New York Academy of Sciences, 1141*(1), 105–130. https://doi.org/10.1196/annals.1441.030

Stone, B. (2022). Positive psychology for substance use disorders: A rationale and call to action. *Journal of Studies on Alcohol and Drugs, 83*(6), 959–961. https://doi.org/10.15288/jsad.22-00259

Tougas, M. E., Hayden, J. A., McGrath, P. J., Huguet, A., & Rozario, S. (2015). A systematic review exploring the social cognitive theory of self-regulation as a framework for chronic health condition interventions. *PLoS One, 10*(8), e134977. https://doi.org/10.1371/journal.pone.0134977

US Department of Health and Human Services (USHHS). (2020). Public health services. Office of the surgeon general. *Smoking cessation: A report of the surgeon general*. Rockville, MD.

Velten, J., Lavallee, K. L., Scholten, S., Meyer, A. H., Zhang, X.-C., Schneider, S., & Margraf, J. (2014). Lifestyle choices and mental health: A representative population survey. *BMC Psychol, 2*(1), 58. https://doi.org/10.1186/s40359-014-0055-y

Vidrine, J. I., Spears, C. A., & Heppner, W. L., Reitzel, L. R., Marcus, M. T., Cinciripini, P. M., Waters, A. J., Li, Y., Nguyen, N. T., Cao Y., Tindle, H. A., Fine, M., Safranek, L. V. & Wetter, D. W. (2016). Efficacy of mindfulness-based addiction treatment (MBAT) for smoking cessation and lapse recovery: A randomized clinical trial. *J Consult Clin Psychol, 84*(9), 824–838. https://doi.org/10.1037/ccp0000117

Vinci, C. (2020). Cognitive-behavioral and mindfulness intervention for smoking cessation: A review of the recent literature. *Current Onc Reports, 22*, Article number 58. https://doi.org/10.1007/s11912-020-00915-w

Vinci, C., Li, L., Wu, C., Lam, C. Y., Guo, L, Correa-Fernandez, V., Spears, C. A., Hoover, D. S., Etchberry, P. E., Wetter, W. D. (2017). The association of positive emotion and first smoking lapse: An ecological monetary assessment study. *Health Psychology, 36*(11), 1038–1046. https://doi.org/10.1037/hea0000535

Wellenzohn, S., Proyer, R. T., & Ruch, W. (2016). Humor-based online positive psychology interventions: A randomized placebo-controlled long-term trial. *The Journal of Positive Psychology, 11*(6), 584–594. https://doi.org/10.1080/17439760. 2015.1137624

Witkiewitz, K., Lustyk, M. K., & Bowen, S. (2013). Retraining the addicted brain: A review of hypothesized neurobiological mechanisms of mindfulness-based relapse prevention. *Psychology of Addictive Behaviors, 27*(2), 351–365. https://doi.org/ 10.1037/a0029258

Witkiewitz, K., Marlatt, G. A., & Walker, D. (2005). Mindfulness-based relapse prevention for alcohol and substance use disorders. *Journal of Cognitive Psychotherapy, 19*(3), 211–228.

Zand, A., Shams, J., Shakeri, N., & Chatr-Zarrin, F. (2017). The relationship between wellbeing and substance abuse relapse. Research in medicine. *Journal of Research in Medical Sciences, 41*(1), 31–36.

Zemansky, T. R. (2006). The risen phoenix: Psychological transformation within the context of long-term sobriety in alcoholics anonymous. *Dissertation Abstracts International: Section B: The Sciences and Engineering, 66*(8-B), 4506. Accessed August 25, 2023. https://search-ebscohost-com.elib.tcd.ie/login.aspx?direct=true& db=psyh&AN=2006-99004-062&site=ehost-live

Zimbardo, P., Sword, R., & Sword, R. (2012). *The time cure: Overcoming PTSD with the new psychology of time perspective therapy.* Jossey-Bass.

7 Positive Psychology in Stress Management

Chapter Overview

This chapter provides a brief overview of the science of positive psychology in managing stress. We introduce practical clinical coaching applications of the PERMA model and other positive psychology interventions (PPIs) to help patients manage their stress. When the stress response is reduced, mental and physical health improve, negative emotions decrease, and positive emotions increase, which support the other healthy lifestyle pillars.

Introduction

Managing stress is a major pillar of a healthy lifestyle. Stress, not only can lead to harmful physiologic consequences (O'Connor et al., 2021), but also plays a role in motivating unhealthy behaviors (Britz & Pappas, 2010; Heuel & Lübstorf, 2022) and stress coping is associated with better multiple health behaviors (Hirooka et al., 2022). Therefore, positive psychology interventions (PPIs) may be considered an essential part of a healthy lifestyle plan, as they have been shown to help counter stress (Hendriks et al., 2020; Moskowitz et al., 2012).

These interventions increase positive emotions that lead to resilience – the ability to adapt to changing situations and setbacks (Southwick et al., 2014) and improve physical health and cognitive function (Fredrickson, 2009). Positive emotions can be especially important in adverse situations to buffer significant stress with greater protective effects on mortality. However, an analysis of datasets from the National Health and Nutrition Examination Survey (NHANES I) and National Health Epidemiological Study (NHEFS) found that the association between positive affect and mortality risk was weaker and not significant among participants who reported low levels of stress (Oakley et al., 2017).

DOI: 10.4324/9781003428909-7

Stress Mindset

However, stress levels are not the only thing that matters. The perception of stress impacts patients' health and wellbeing. In a study with 28,753 US adults, the researchers explored the amount of stress they experienced over 12 months (Keller et al., 2012). They ranged from a lot of stress to none at all. Additionally, participants were asked to assess how much stress they believed affected their health, with some participants claiming it impacted them a lot, hardly, or not at all. Eight years later, the researchers sampled the National Death Index to identify participants' mortality rates. Those who reported a lot of stress and perceived stress as adversely impacting their health increased their risk of premature death during this time by 43%. Those who experienced no stress or hardly any stress but believed that stress was bad for them reported a 10% increase in premature death. The lowest incidence of premature death was reported by individuals who experienced a lot of stress but did not believe it impacted their health negatively. Their risk of prematurely dying was barely 8% despite living a stressful life for at least a year. This research was the first one to show that the impact of stress depends, not only on the amount of stress we experience but also on our attitude toward it.

Our negative attitude toward stress stems from its biased portrayal in the media. It is perceived as harmful, and we were taught to be alert, fear the consequences of stress, and find strategies to calm down. As such, as soon as our heart starts racing, we practice breathing techniques or positive affirmations to calm it down. Stress symptoms have become an unwanted part of our daily lives, and we have learned to fear them and see them as harming our health. But what if our attitude toward stress changes? What if we start differentiating stress from distress and stop fearing the symptoms?

Here is an alternative way of perceiving stress. When facing a stressor, our liver dumps fat and sugar into the bloodstream for fuel. Our breathing deepens so that more oxygen is delivered to our hearts. Our heart rate speeds up to deliver oxygen, fat, and sugar to our muscles and brain to support us in thinking of a solution to our problem or running away from danger. Our body creates this stress reaction to help us, not hinder us.

What we do with this whole-body activation is up to us. When individuals become conditioned by the media to fear this state of alert, they tend to ignore the symptoms or focus all their attention on calming themselves. They do it by breathing deeper, counting to ten, or sometimes, they use substances, such as alcohol, tobacco, or drugs, to help them. Focused on the symptoms, they ignore the source of stress.

However, those no longer conditioned to perceive their stress as unfavorable see it as a resource that enhances their performance. This way, when they begin to experience the symptoms of stress, instead of searching for ways to get rid of the uncomfortable feeling stress creates in their bodies, they focus their attention on gathering social resources to help them tackle their issues or getting to the root of the problem that causes the stress reaction. The coping strategies they use are diametrically different from those of a group that fears stress, and as such, their health and wellbeing outcomes differ. These two attitudes toward stress are called "stress mindsets" (Crum et al., 2017). They are an additional and essential variable that impacts our experiences of stress. They differ significantly from cognitive reappraisals and coping strategies (Silva et al., 2023). Given that we can control them, sometimes more so than the amount of stress we experience in life, they are a valuable resource that needs to be considered when exploring stress management techniques. Instead of focusing on appraising the stressor as more or less stressful, stress mindset appraises the nature of stress as enhancing (stress is helpful) or debilitating (stress is harmful). For example, when an individual is experiencing a stressful diagnosis-waiting period that they cannot control, they can view the stress they experience as harmful, meaning they expect it to impact their health and vitality negatively. Alternatively, they can view it as helpful, whereby the stress they experience will result in higher levels of resilience, experiences of posttraumatic growth, or an ability to connect with people who can support them sincerely.

In the last decade, an avalanche of research has helped us understand the impact of stress mindsets on health and wellbeing beyond decreased mortality. Viewing stress as enhancing acts as a buffer against stress, making individuals more likely to use more effective coping strategies and perceive stress as less threatening (Jenkins et al., 2021). As such, in a group of highly stressed college students, a stress-is-enhancing mindset mitigated their symptoms of depression and anxiety a month later, thus improving their coping (Huebschmann & Sheets, 2020). Furthermore, a stress-is-enhancing mindset predicted psychological wellbeing and significantly lowered somatic symptoms of stress (Keech et al., 2020). Emerging evidence suggests it is also associated with better cardiovascular health (Hendricks et al., 2023). It increases anabolic (growth) hormones, improves physiological health, and protects against higher cortisol awakening response (Silva et al., 2023). Thus, from the health point of view, a stress-is-enhancing mindset is correlated with better physiological, physical, and psychological health and wellbeing.

During the COVID-19 pandemic, healthcare professionals with a stress-is-enhancing mindset reported higher levels of posttraumatic growth compared to those with a stress-is-debilitating mindset (Zhang et al., 2023). Their growth happened as a result of engaging in more proactive coping behaviors. Furthermore, research with nurses showed that a stress-is-enhancing mindset was directly related to resilience and indirectly related to mental health (Emirza & Yılmaz, 2023). Introducing healthier stress mindsets to healthcare professionals can help them cope more effectively with the daily stress associated with the workplace. Finally, individuals with a healthy stress mindset are also less judgemental about their colleagues experiencing heavy workloads (Ben-Avi et al., 2018); their stress-related attitude can facilitate better teamwork. All these benefits can be accomplished by engaging in various interventions that support healthy mindsets.

Two types of interventions have been developed to help change mindsets: stress reappraisal and stress mindset (Jamieson et al., 2018). The reappraisal relates to acknowledging stress responses as functional, seeing stress as a resource, and using it for active coping. The stress mindset interventions involve acknowledging positive and negative aspects of stress, welcoming and utilizing stress to enhance performance. These interventions result in individuals paying less attention to the negative emotional stimuli; it improves their cognitive flexibility, thus allowing them to rethink their options. It also motivates them to make a change and perceive more resources, all of which result in improved performance, a higher level of wellbeing, and persistence in accomplishing what is important to them.

Given that the stress mindset is modifiable, various interventions have been applied to change it. Most of the interventions have focused on educating participants about the positive impact of stress. They included short videos (three minutes) or paragraphs sharing research showing the positive effects of stress or feeling anxious. However, recently, a metacognitive approach to changing mindsets was introduced, offering a balanced appraisal of stress, i.e., acknowledging stress's positive and negative impact (Crum et al., 2023). This resulted in greater physiological health outcomes beyond discussing only the positive impact of stress. Thus, for best results, we need to consider both.

Stanford Rethinking Stress Tools

Access rethinking stress tools free of charge online: https://sparqtools.org/rethinkingstress/. The Stanford SPARQ (Social Psychological Answers to Real-World Questions) tools offer a range of videos the aim of which is to change mindsets.

The activities include thinking about a time when you performed at your highest level and reflecting on what fuelled your high performance. It is about reframing stress and considering not only what stresses you now, but also why it stresses you, from the perspective of what you care about that impacts your higher stress levels.

Passion and Stress

Passion for an activity or work fuels our lives, making them worthwhile. Frequently, passionate physicians and nurses get the best out of their love for work but may pay for it with health issues such as burnout. It is because not all types of passions are good for us. According to the dualistic model of passion

(Vallerand et al., 2003), passion helps us improve our performance and success; however, depending on whether it is harmonious or obsessive, it can either improve or negatively impact our wellbeing.

Our internal mechanisms drive harmonious passion (Carpentier et al., 2012). We engage in an activity because we enjoy it or it fulfills us. We focus on the positive emotions the work helps us experience and how it makes us feel at our best. Thus, we do our passionate activity to sustain these feelings. After completing an activity, we can experience psychological flow in this and other aspects of our lives. Flow is that feeling when we lose ourselves in an activity to the extent that we are unaware of the time, place, or people around us. The flow requires focus and challenge, so while in flow, we might not feel happy; however, we are flooded with endorphins afterward. They leave us feeling content and wanting more of that positive boost.

Obsessive passion, on the other hand, is driven by external factors. We do our work as we seek recognition and promotion or feel externally pressured because other people have high expectations of us. We engage in obsessively passionate work to avoid negative emotions. For example, some individuals who train for a marathon feel guilty when they sit at home relaxing, or workaholics feel guilty when they spend time with family and friends. Thus, to avoid the negative emotions, they keep training and working and feel like they cannot help themselves. The passion controls them, and they feel obliged to keep going.

Both groups of people are successful at achieving their goals. However, while harmoniously passionate people practice healthy flexibility when pursuing their goals, obsessively passionate people keep up with their rigid persistence, no matter what, for which they pay with health and wellbeing. For example, in a landmark study, a group of ballerinas who sustained injuries were compared for their passion. Those with harmonious passion consulted with their physicians sooner than the obsessively passionate ballerinas; they spent more time resting after an injury and tended to engage in more strict self-initiated injury prevention techniques (Rip et al., 2006). Subsequently, the obsessive ballerinas experienced prolonged suffering from chronic injuries as they continued to dance despite injury, meaning that their bodies had not healed properly, which further resulted in their poorer health outcomes. Thus, regarding health and wellbeing, obsessive passion leads to unwise decisions.

Because of the pressure obsessively passionate people put upon themselves, they tend to experience more stress (Zhou, 2021). Furthermore, while they might be able to experience psychological flow, which is associated with improved wellbeing, their flow is limited to passionate activity (Carpentier et al., 2012; Lavigne et al., 2012). When engaging in another activity, they ruminate about their favorite activity to such an extent that it reduces their subjective wellbeing and flows into other experiences. On the other hand, harmoniously passionate people can enjoy various activities without rumination. They can stay in the present moment for all of them.

The most significant difference between the obsessively and harmoniously passionate people is wellbeing. Obsessive passion leads to lower engagement (Birkland & Buch, 2015), lower life satisfaction (Thorgren et al., 2013), higher anxiety, depression, burnout (Vallerand et al., 2010), and emotional exhaustion (Fernet et al., 2014). To date, little is known of specific interventions that can be used to help individuals experience harmonious passion. Usually, awareness of the type of passion that we are driven by can help people make changes to more adaptive and helpful to their wellbeing. Another way to do this is via character strengths (Forest et al., 2012). Individuals who engage in character strengths turn their passion from obsessive to harmonious, thus allowing them to enjoy the work they do and experience less stress.

Applications of Positive Psychology for Stress Management

Research investigating specific interventions to increase positive emotions and manage stress has included a range of constructs, including gratitude, mindfulness, social support, and cognitive behavioral therapy (CBT). In a highly-cited gratitude study (Emmons & McCullough, 2003), participants who wrote down things they were grateful for every day experienced an increase in positive emotions and a decrease in negative emotions, such as reactions to stressful situations. Mindfulness-based stress reduction (MBSR) by paying attention to the present moment without judgment is a well-known technique (Kabat-Zin, 2013) shown to be effective in reducing stress and increasing positive emotions. Flow exercises or activities – which can lead to being fully present with an activity – may also be recommended as stress relievers. Social support resources provided by family, friends, and even pets, in the form of emotional support, advice, and assistance can buffer the negative effects of stress on physical and mental health (Cohen & Wills, 1985). CBT is also a key tool for managing stress in both clinical and general populations (Nakao et al., 2021).

Of particular relevance to positive health approaches is the finding that multiple-component positive affect interventions (MMPIs) – combinations of these kinds of PPIs – have also been shown to both increase positive affect and decrease negative affect. Hence, MMPIS, which is found useful to address stress, is recommended as part of a lifestyle plan for coping with and buffering against stress (Moskowitz et al., 2012).

Positive psychology principles can be applied in various ways for managing stress. One technique is writing about life goals. Study participants who wrote about their life goals experienced a decrease in stress and an increase in wellbeing (King, 2001). This technique can be effective when the writing focuses on their strengths and values that lead to a greater sense of self-efficacy and purpose. Loving-kindness meditation practice, which involves directing positive emotions toward oneself and others (Fredrickson, 2013) can also increase positive emotions, social connectedness, and wellbeing. PPIs for stress are being tested in specific populations, such as women workers (Santos et al., 2021).

In reference to one of the stress-reducing positive psychology techniques noted above that involves writing about strengths and values, we need to highlight another writing technique that, although not a positive psychology one per se, is often discussed in the context of stress-induced from trauma. Individuals who have experienced trauma may derive mental health benefits by expressing negative emotions in the context of writing a coherent story (Pennebaker, 1993). Analysis of the writings shows a reduction of negative emotions in the process of writing (Tonarelli et al, 2017). Despite several meta-analyses validating the expressive writing intervention (Gerger et al, 2022), results have been mixed; for example, one meta-analysis showed no significant effect on health (Mogk et al., 2006). A recent study found a reduction in psychological distress among asymptomatic COVID-19 patients (Zheng et al., 2022). Therefore, to help address stress in the context of trauma, expressive writing may be considered and enhanced with positive psychology constructs by also writing about strengths, values, and goals.

Expressive Writing (Pennebaker & Evans, 2014)

The basic instruction for this activity is to sit and write for 15–20 minutes about your deepest thoughts and feelings associated with an upsetting or traumatic situation. The objective of this is not to resolve anything, but rather express yourself the best way you can without judgment. The more meaningful and thoughtful the writing, the more impact it has on wellbeing. Most importantly, please do not worry about any spelling mistakes. You will not be reading back what you are writing, just externalizing what's inside of you.

In case you get stuck in your expressive writing, researchers offer several strategies to get unstuck. Here are some options:

- Sit down in front of the mirror and write. Every now and then, look at your mirror image to remind you to be honest about yourself.
- Think about a specific audience, e.g. your friends. What would your friends think when they see you write this?
- Start with a "stream-of-consciousness" writing, i.e. I'm sitting here and do not really know what to write about...
- Re-write your traumatic situation into a story.
- Write from various perspectives, e.g. when it is difficult to write about what happened to you, write from the third person perspective (she, he), then change to the second person (you) and then to the first person writing (I). Similarly, you can write from the bigger perspective (the world), moderate perspective (your family), or minute perspective (yourself).

Everyone has a different time of day for improving the effectiveness of this activity. Some prefer to write in the morning, others at lunchtime, before bedtime, or in the middle of the night, if they cannot sleep and something weighs on their mind. It is important that individuals find your their time and form of expression. While writing is useful for many, some prefer to use other media, such as a smartphone recorder, video, or visual arts.

In addition to expressive writing, we can also put a positive psychology twist on self-expression by exploring positive topics in our writing. Doing so impacts our stress levels via a range of processes, including positive reappraisal or experiences of positive emotions.

Benefit-finding is one such approach. It recognizes that finding benefits in dire situations is a way for people to adapt to changed circumstances and manage stress (Tennen & Affleck, 2005). In a landmark study with mothers whose children were acutely ill, citing at least one benefit of their desperate situation predicted less distress and improved mood between 6 and 18 months later (Affleck et al., 1991). It is common for people who experience distress to find benefits in it at some stage of the adjustment process and often it happens approximately 12–18 months after the event (Tennen & Affleck, 2005). To facilitate this natural process, we can conduct this activity soon after the traumatic event has occurred. In one study cancer patients were asked to write about benefits over four sessions and the results showed that their physical symptoms and medical appointments declined compared to the control group (Stanton, Danoff-Burg, & Sworowski, 2002). In another study, those who engaged in a benefit-writing activity showed a significant reduction in doctor visits for up to three months and an improvement in health and wellbeing for up to five months (King & Miner, 2000).

Benefits Finding (King & Miner, 2000)

Recall a traumatic life event or some loss you have experienced in your life. Think about the experience for a few moments. Now, focus on the positive aspects of the experience. Please write about how you have personally changed or grown as a result of the experience. Focus on the positive aspects and how the experience has benefited you as a person – how has the experience made you better able to meet the challenges of the future? As you write, do not worry about punctuation or grammar, just really let go and write as much as you can about the positive aspects of the experience.

An eight-week multicomponent program was developed for older adults and showed an increase in a happiness, life satisfaction, reduction in perceived stress and depression (Turner et al., 2017). Its content was based on positive psychological research and included in-class activities as well as homework. Throughout the program, participants were introduced to what constituted happiness. They were encouraged to reflect on what makes them happy, explore the concept of compassion and gratitude and discuss the causes of stress and stress management techniques. They also familiarized themselves with the importance of forgiveness as a foundation for wellbeing and ways in which they can transform self-created suffering, such as guilt and blame, into a positive experience. Finally, the program helped participants develop mindfulness and develop a sense of humor as a coping strategy.

Selected "Homework" Activities from The Art of Happiness Program (Adapted from Turner et al., 2012)

Letters of Forgiveness

1 Write a letter to someone whom you treated unfairly. In your letter, you can either apologize for your actions or offer them forgiveness.
2 Write a letter of apology to yourself for something you should not have done in the past and which you regret doing.
3 Write a letter of forgiveness to someone who has hurt you in the past.

Savoring

Using a small piece of fruit or any other type of healthy food, let it melt in your mouth or chew slowly, noticing flavors, textures and chewing sounds you have not noticed before.

Prospecting

Each morning, write down three things that you look forward to that day and then at the end of the day, write down three things that went well for you that day. Repeat this activity as frequently as you wish.

Using Strengths at Your Personal Best (Adapted from Forest et al., 2012)

Write down or speak to a friend about you at your personal best. Describe how you work, what you do, and how it feels when you are at your personal best.

Now complete a free Virtues in Action (VIA)character survey (www. viacharacter.org), identify your five top strengths, and write down what it would be like if you used your strengths doing what you do when you're at your personal best.

Finally, select two of your strengths and use them in a novel way over the next week.

Positive Psychology for Reducing Stress in Individuals with Physical or Mental Illness

Key positive psychology skills that can help manage stress among individuals with serious illnesses, such as HIV and metastatic breast cancer, affective disorders, drug addiction, and caregiving include noticing, savoring or planning positive experiences, improving relationships, and pursuing meaningful or personal development goals. Positive affect interventions can be taught while avoiding dismissing negative affect that can help bring attention to needed self-care (Saslow et al., 2014).

A systematic review of 50 randomized controlled trials found that multi-component PPIs were effective in improving subjective wellbeing, depression, psychological wellbeing, anxiety, and stress. However, the limited number of studies on anxiety and stress precluded definitive conclusions, and further studies were recommended for diverse populations (Hendriks et al., 2020). More research is also needed to identify which PPIs are effective in different populations.

PERMA for Managing Stress

As we've seen with other healthy lifestyle pillars, the PERMA framework can be harnessed in the process of managing stress. Below is an outline of PERMA questions related to stress one could consider for identifying action steps.

Application of PERMA in the Context of Stress Management

P—Positive emotions: Do activities that increase positive feelings during a stressful time.
- What kinds of activities bring forth calming feelings when you have a stressful time?
- How can you help yourself to pay attention to relaxing and positive experiences or memories when you feel stressed?

E—Engagement (Flow): Do activities that get you fully immersed in them, such as making art, playing music, dancing, and gardening, during stressful times.

- What activities have given you a sense of flow and that you can do during stressful times?
- What new activities would you like to try that could produce a sense of flow even during stressful times?

R—Relationships: Identify how you can increase positive social interactions.

- What are social activities you could engage in during stressful times?
- Who can you connect with positively for support during stressful times?

M—Meaning: Pay attention to the things in your life that are meaningful to you.

- What are meaningful activities you can do when you are feeling stressed?
- How does taking action to protect and improve your wellbeing in the face of difficult and stressful times add to your life purpose and sense of meaning?

A—Achievement: Notice and celebrate any progress you are making toward goals that are important to you, including taking action to buffer yourself against the effects of stress.

- What activities have you accomplished or made progress on that make you feel proud?
- What small steps have you achieved toward your stress management goal?

Appreciative Inquiry to Support Stress Management

Appreciative inquiry can be used in developing an action plan that boosts positive emotions and leverages character and other personal strengths to help counter the emotional and physical consequences of stress.

Discovery: What are you doing now to manage stress?

- What are the positive habits that help you during stressful times?
- What activities do you do now or have done recently that boost your positive emotions and counter negative reactions to stress, e.g. hanging out with friends?
- Which personal strengths do you use when faced with stressful situations?

Dream: What changes are possible that create joy and other positive feelings to balance out stress reactions?

- What activities that bring joy and counter negative stress reactions are possible?

- What changes are possible that build one's capacity to stay calm and positive during stressful times?

Design: What positive changes could you make that build your capacity to manage your emotions and behaviors, and even thrive, during stressful times?
- What is your favorite positive activity that you could build into your lifestyle habits during stressful times?
- How could you use your personal strengths to counter negative reactions to stress?

Destiny: What positive changes are you confident you can make to support you during stressful times?
- What positive activity action plan are you ready to make to increase a sense of calm, joy, pride, and other positive feelings, even during stressful times?
- Which personal strengths are you confident you will rely on to achieve your stress management action plan?
- What are healthy ways to reward yourself as you make progress toward your action plan?

Positive Psychology in the Lifestyle Medicine Competencies: Emotional and Mental Health Assessments and Interventions

As with the other lifestyle medicine pillars, positive psychology can be integrated into lifestyle medicine competencies. Health providers can adopt well-known models of positive psychology, such as PERMA and appreciative inquiry into clinical practice. The lifestyle medicine competencies in the area of mental and emotional health can particularly benefit from an enhanced application of positive psychology principles and approaches. Below are suggested positive psychology expansions for several of these competencies.

- While applying screening tools for stress, depression, and anxiety in clinical practice, also use screening tools for assessing positive emotions and life satisfaction, which can be harnessed for stress management.
- When explaining the relationship and pathophysiology between emotional and physical health, include the physiological benefits of positive emotions.
- In describing and utilizing evidence-based and patient-centered mental and emotional health, including self-management and resilience-building techniques, also describe and utilize PPIs as essential self-care tools and stress intervention techniques.
- When analyzing the clinical relevance and evidence base for MBSR and related stress management strategies, include the evidence base for PPIs on stress management.
- In treatment plans for lifestyle-related mental health diseases, such as depression and anxiety, apply PPIs as primary or supplementary treatments.

Table 7.1 Integrating positive health into lifestyle medicine competencies: Emotional and mental health assessments and interventions

Lifestyle medicine competencies	Positive health expansion
Apply screening tools for stress, depression, and anxiety in clinical practice	While screening for negative emotions and mental illness, include assessment for positive emotions and life satisfaction that can be harnessed for stress management
Explain the relationship and pathophysiology between emotional and physical health	Explain the physiological benefits of positive emotions
Describe and utilize evidence-based and patient-centered mental and emotional health, including self-management and resilience-building techniques	Describe and utilize PPIs as essential self-care tools and stress intervention techniques
Analyze the clinical relevance and evidence base for MBSR and related stress management strategies	Analyze the evidence base for PPIs on stress management
Manage treatment plans for lifestyle-related mental health diseases, such as depression and anxiety	Manage treatment plans with PPIs as primary or supplementary treatments
Apply mindfulness skills to enable presence, clarity, and curiosity in the clinical encounter	Along with mindfulness skills, role model positive psychology approaches for patients during the clinical encounter, such as asking what has gone well for them recently

- In addition to applying mindfulness skills to enable presence, clarity, and curiosity in the clinical encounter, role model positive psychology approaches for patients, such as asking what has gone well for them recently.

Table 7.1 shows the lifestyle medicine competencies for emotional and mental health assessment and interventions in the left column and suggests expansions of these competencies for a positive health practice in the right column.

Perspectives in Practicing from the Inside Out – Stress Management

In addition to traditional methods of stress management of breathing and mindfulness practices, positive psychology approaches are often used for managing stress in self-care and health care. These strategies have also been applied in positive psychiatry as part of mental illness treatment and other settings. Health coaches, health providers, and other health team members consider applying PPIs in the context of stress, because such activities may naturally counter negative feelings, such as anxiety in the face of difficulties. The lifestyle medicine pillars are interconnected and, therefore, positive psychology can be harnessed for managing stress while advancing a comprehensive healthy lifestyle treatment and health maintenance plan.

As the health team engages with the individual about PPIs for stress, think about how these interventions can also influence the other pillars in a positive way, particularly in helping to nudge health behavior changes. Positive psychology approaches can be powerful for stressed individuals in that they have the potential to directly improve psychological wellbeing, reduce physical risk factors, enhance health protective factors, and support successful health behavior changes. All of this can help balance out the negative consequences of stress, as well as promote overall wellbeing.

In some cases, high levels of stress and other emotional and mental health conditions can interfere with making progress toward a healthy lifestyle. Addressing these barriers first needs to become a priority. Letting go of the immediate goal to facilitate healthy eating and physical activity, for example, the practitioner might need to focus on one or two small steps the individual can take to create feelings of calm and joy that may get them unstuck to pursue a healthy lifestyle.

The practitioner can apply positive psychology techniques in a compassionate manner that acknowledges the patient's negative experiences and difficult circumstances and takes into account their history, cultural background, and current environment. It's crucial that the patient feels understood and that their current "survival" habits are honored, despite how maladaptive and unhealthy those behaviors may be. From that place of understanding and connection, we can touch on the elements of PERMA or conduct an appreciative inquiry interview to identify even one small positive step to serve as the crystal core for moving forward toward self-care and healthy habits in the face of challenges and major stress.

Positive Psychology Clinical Approaches and Tools to Address Stress

As we've seen a wide array of PPIs and approaches can be leveraged to help patients address high levels of stress. These approaches can be incorporated into prescriptions.

Example of a Positive Psychology Stress Management Prescription

Identify one character strength you can use in managing your stress. Apply it regularly.

Each week, write down how you have used that character strength and note your progress in lowering your stressed feelings.

Refills: Continue this process with your other strengths

Use sharing, strengths, and savoring to support your stress management goal:

Sharing – When feeling stressed, reach out to a family member or friend for support; they can remind you to lean on your strengths.

Strengths – This is built into the prescription.

Savoring – Savor positive feelings when applying your strengths to feel more in control under stressful situations.

Example of an Action Plan

"I will use my strengths of forgiveness and kindness to help me through my stressful time at work. I will think about how my coworkers and my boss are human and may also be struggling and forgive them for their requests and actions that seem unreasonable. I will write down my progress every Saturday morning."

Case Study of Positive Health Approaches for Managing Stress

Patient Background: Sarah, a 35-year-old, overweight project assistant, was diagnosed with type II diabetes two years ago. She has been struggling to manage her blood sugar levels with the lifestyle prescriptions of a mostly plant-based diet and increased activity, as well as the medication, metformin. She feels overwhelmed by the demands of the disease and feels she did not get compassionate care from her last provider. She experiences frequent episodes of stress and anxiety related to her diabetes management, which has been impacting her quality of life.

Assessment: The provider screens for anxiety and depression. She determines that Sarah has a high level of stress, but does not meet the criteria for depression and is not suicidal. The provider also assesses Sarah's life satisfaction using the Satisfaction with Life Scale, which results in a score of 18, indicating that Sarah needs activities to boost her life satisfaction.

Intervention: The provider suggests that she try using positive psychology techniques to manage her stress, before focusing on her current eating and physical activity habits. The diabetes educator conducts a review of the PERMA elements and helps Sarah identify that she is interested in trying mindfulness meditation. She had signed up for a meditation class to manage her stress in college, but she had only been able to attend for a few weeks before her schedule got in the way.

She recalls liking the calm feelings she experienced during the guided meditations.

Action Plan: Sarah sets a goal that she feels is achievable of doing mindful breathing for 15 minutes every other morning. She plans to reward herself each week that she achieves her goal with a trip to visit a friend. The diabetes educator encourages her to make sure to seek social support on days she is not able to see her friend.

Progress: Sarah also works with a diabetes educator on her self-talk to counteract negative thoughts about her diabetes. Instead of viewing this condition as a burden, she is learning to reframe it as an opportunity to take care of herself better and prioritize her wellbeing. A couple of weeks later, she added gratitude practice to her action plan, by spending a few minutes each Saturday to focus on the positive aspects of her life, especially the support she receives from her sister and healthcare team.

Outcome: After a couple of months of meditation and gratitude practices and reframing her self-talk, Sarah begins to feel more in control of her negative emotions, stress, and anxiety. She becomes more confident that she can make progress with her eating and physical activity treatment plan that had been recommended while enjoying a more balanced and fulfilling life.

Key Take-Aways: Positive psychology techniques can be an effective way to manage stress in individuals with diabetes and other chronic conditions requiring significant lifestyle changes. By bringing attention to what is going well, their strengths, and their accomplishments, individuals can develop a more positive outlook on their medical disease treatment plan and thrive despite the challenges of making significant lifestyle changes.

Conclusion

Awareness of the impact of varying levels of stress, the different outcomes of stress mindsets (whether stress is perceived as positive or negative), and the relationship of obsessive passion to stress can spur insights for creating effective stress management. Positive psychology offers a unique approach to addressing stress through a focus on building habits that lead to resilience and personal growth in the face of stress and promoting positive health and wellbeing.

By cultivating positive emotions and doing positive activities routinely, including social support, individuals can improve their ability to manage daily stressors and major adverse events. The health team can nudge behavior change for proactive stress management by asking questions based on the PERMA framework, conducting appreciative inquiry focused on stress, and making PPI prescriptions. Techniques such as gratitude, mindfulness, and loving-kindness meditation can be effective in buffering against negative physiologic responses and illness and promoting positive emotions despite life's adversities. PPIs can be applied to healthy living in self-care, in various community settings, including schools, workplaces, and healthcare settings, to help individuals manage their stress, lead more fulfilling lives, and achieve positive health.

References

Affleck, G., Tennen, H., & Rowe, J. (1991). Infants in crisis: How parents cope with newborn intensive care and its aftermath. Springer-Verlag Publishing/Springer Nature. https://doi-org.elib.tcd.ie/10.1007/978-1-4612-3050-2

Ben-Avi, N., Toker, S., & Heller, D. (2018). "If stress is good for me, it's probably good for you too": Stress mindset and judgment of others' strain. *Journal of Experimental Social Psychology, 74*, 98–110. https://doi.org/10.1016/j.jesp.2017.09.002

Birkland, I. K., & Buck, R. (2015). The dualistic model of passion for work: Discriminate and predictive validity with work engagement and workaholism. *Motivation and Emotion. 39*(3), 392–408. https://doi.org/10.1007/s11031-014-9462-x.

Britz, J., & Pappas, E. (2010). Sources and outlets of stress among university students: Correlations between stress and unhealthy habits. *Undergraduate Research Journal for the Human Sciences, 9*.

Carpentier, J., Mageau, G. A., & Vallerand, R. J. (2012). Ruminations and flow: Why do people with a more harmonious passion experience higher well-being? *Journal of Happiness Studies: An Interdisciplinary Forum on Subjective Well-Being, 13*(3), 501–518. https://doi.org/10.1007/s10902-011-9276-4.

Cohen, S., & Wills, T. A. (1985). Stress, social support, and the buffering hypothesis. *Psychological Bulletin, 98*(2), 310–357.

Crum, A. J., Santoro, E., Handley-Miner, I., Smith, E. N., Evans, K., Moraveji, N., Achor, S., & Salovey, P. (2023). Evaluation of the "rethink stress" mindset intervention: A metacognitive approach to changing mindsets. *Journal of Experimental Psychology: General, 152*(9), 2603–2622. https://doi.org/10.1037/xge0001396.

Emirza, S., & Yılmaz Kozcu, G. (2023). Protecting healthcare workers' mental health against COVID-19-related stress: The effects of stress mindset and psychological resilience. *Nursing & Health Sciences, 25*(2), 216–230. https://doi.org/10.1111/nhs. 13018.

Emmons, R. A., & McCullough (2003). Counting blessings versus burdens: An experimental investigation of gratitude and subjective well-being in daily life. *Journal of Personality and Social Psychology, 84*(2), 377–389. https://doi.org/10.1037/0022-3514.84.2.377.

Fernet, C., Lavigne, G. L., Vallerand, R. J., & Austin, S. (2014). Fired up with passion: Investigating how job autonomy and passion predict burnout at career start in teachers. *Work & Stress, 28*(3), 270–288. https://doi.org/10.1080/02678373.2014.935524.

Forest, J., Mageau, G. A., Crevier-Braud, L., Bergeron, É, Dubreuil, P., & Lavigne, G. L. (2012). Harmonious passion as an explanation of the relation between signature strengths' use and well-being at work: Test of an intervention program. *Human Relations, 65*(9), 1233–1252. https://doi.org/10.1177/0018726711433134.

Fredrickson, B. L. (2009). *Positivity*. Crown Publishers.

Fredrickson, B. L. (2013). Positive emotions broaden and build. In S. J. Lopez & C. R. Snyder (Eds.), *Oxford handbook of positive psychology* (2nd ed., pp. 129–143). Oxford University Press.

Gerger, H., Werner, C. P., Gaab, J., & Culipers, P. (2022). Comparative efficacy and acceptability of expressive writing treatments compared to other writing treatments, and waiting list control for adult trauma survivors: A systematic review and network meta-analysis. *Psychological Medicine, 52*(15), 3484–3496. https://doi.org/10.1017/S0033291721000143.

Hendricks, B., Quinn, T. D., Price, B. S., Dotson, T., Claydon, E. A., & Miller, R. (2023). Impact of stress and stress mindset on prevalence of cardiovascular disease risk factors among first responders. *BMC Public Health, 23*(1), 1–8. https://doi.org/10.1186/s12889-023-16819-w.

Hendriks, T., Schotanus-Dijkstra, M., & Hassankhan, A. de Jong, J., & Bohlmeijer, E. (2020). The efficacy of multi-component positive psychology interventions: A systematic review and meta-analysis of randomized controlled trials. *Journal of Happiness Studies, 21*(1), 357–390. https://doi.org/10.1007/s10902-019-00082-1

Heuel, L., & Lübstorf, S. (2022). Chronic stress, behavioral tendencies, and determinants of health behaviors in nurses: A mixed-methods approach. *BMC Public Health, 22.* https://doi.org/10.1186/s12889-022-12993-5

Hirooka, N., Kusano, T., Kinoshita, S., & Nakamoto, H. (2022). Influence of perceived stress and stress coping adequacy on multiple health-related lifestyle behaviors. *International Journal of Environmental Research and Public Health, 19*(1), 284. https://doi.org/10.3390/ijerph19010284.

Huebschmann, N. A., & Sheets, E. S. (2020). The right mindset: Stress mindset moderates the association between perceived Stress and depressive symptoms. *Anxiety, Stress, and Coping, 33*(3), 248–255. https://doi.org/10.1080/10615806.2020.1736900.

Jamieson, J. P., Crum, A. J., Goyer, J. P., Marotta, M. E., & Akinola, M. (2018). Optimizing stress responses with reappraisal and mindset interventions: an integrated model. *Anxiety Stress Coping, 31*(2), 245–261. https://doi.org/10.1080/10615806.2018.1442615

Jenkins, A., Weeks, M. S., & Hard, B. M. (2021). General and specific stress mindsets: Links with college student health and academic performance. *PLoS ONE, 16*(9). https://doi.org/10.1371/journal.pone.0256351

Kabat-Zin, J. (2013). *Full catastrophe living: Using the wisdom of your body and mind to face stress, pain, and illness.* Bantam.

Keech, J. J., Cole, K. L., Hagger, M. S., & Hamilton, K. (2020). The association between stress mindset and physical and psychological wellbeing: Testing a stress beliefs model in police officers. *Psychology & Health, 35*(11), 1306–1325. https://doi.org/10.1080/08870446.2020.1743841.

Keller, A., Litzelman, K., Wisk, L. E., Maddox, T., Cheng, E. R., Creswell, P. D., & Witt, W. P. (2012). Does the perception that stress affects health matter? The association with health and mortality. *Health Psychology, 31*(5), 677–684. https://doi.org/10.1037/a0026743.

King, L. A. (2001). The health benefits of writing about life goals. *Personality and Social Psychology Bulletin, 27*(7), 798–807. https://doi.org/10.1177/0146167201277003.

King, L.A., & Miner, K. N. (2000). Writing about the perceived benefits of traumatic events: Implications for physical health. *Personality and Social Psychology Bulletin, 26*(2), 220–230. https://doi.org/10.1177/0146167200264008

Lavigne, G. L., Forest, J., & Crevier-Baud, L. (2012). Passion at work and burnout: A two-study test of the meditating role of flow experiences. *European Journal of Work and Organizational Psychology, 21*(4), 518–546. https://doi.org/10.1080/135 9432X.2011.578390

Mogk, C., Otte, S., Reinhold-Hurley, B., & Kröner-Herwig, B. (2006). Health effects of expressive writing on stressful or traumatic experiences – A meta-analysis. *Psychosocial Medicine, 3*, Doc06.

Moskowitz, J. T., Hult, J. R., Duncan, L. G., Cohn, M. A., Maurer, S., Bussolari, C., & Acree, M. (2012). A positive affect intervention for people experiencing health-related stress: Development and non-randomized pilot test. *Journal of Health Psychology, 17*(5), 676–692. https://doi.org/10.1177/1359105311425275.

Nakao, M., Shirotsuki, K., & Sugaya, N. (2021). Cognitive-behavioral therapy for management of mental health and stress-related disorders: Recent advances in techniques and technologies. *Bio Pschyo Social Med, 15*, Article 16.

Oakley, J. A., Weiss, A., & Gale, C. R. (2017). The interaction between stress and positive affect in predicting mortality. *Journal of Psychosomatic Research, 100*, 53–60. https://doi.org/10.1016/j.jpsychores.2017.07.005

O'Connor, D. B., Thayer, J. F., & Vedhara, K. (2021). Stress and health: A review of psychobiological processes. *Annual Review of Psychology, 72*, 663–688. https://doi.org/10.1146/annurev-psych-062520-122331

Pennebaker, J. W. (1993). Putting stress into words: Health, linguistic, and therapeutic implications. *Behaviour Research and Therapy, 31960*, 539–548. https://doi.org/10.1016/0005-7967(93)90105-4

Pennebaker, J. W., & Evans, J. F. (2014). Expressive Writing: Words That Heal. Idyll Arbor, Incorporated.

Rip B., Fortin S., & Vallerand R.J. (2006). The relationship between passion and injury in dance students. Journal of Dance Medicine & Science, 10(1/2), 14–20. https://doi-org.elib.tcd.ie/10.1177/1089313x06010001-205

Santos, F. R. M. D., Lacerda, S. S., & Coelhoso, C. C., Barrichello, C.R., Tobo, P.R., & Kozasa, E.H. (2021). The integration of mediation and positive psychology practices to relieve stress in women workers (flourish): Effects in two pilot studies. *Behavioral Science (Basel), 11*(4), 43.

Saslow, L.R., Cohn, M., & Moskowitz, J. T. (2014). Positive affect interventions to reduce stress: Harnessing the benefit while avoiding the pollyanna. In J. Gruber, & J.T. Moskowitz (Eds.), *Positive emotion: Integrating the light sides and dark Sides* (pp. 515–532). Oxford University Press.

Silva, F. C., Ferrreira, M. T., & Souza-Talarico, J. N. (2023). Mapping stress-mindset definitions, measurements and associated factors: A scope review. *Psychoneuroendocrinology, 153*. https://doi.org/10.1016/j.psyneuen.2023.106227

Southwick, S. M., Bonanno, G. A., Masten, A. S., Panter-Brick, C., & Yehuda, R. (2014). Resilience definitions, theory, and challenges: Interdisciplinary perspectives. *European Journal of Psychotraumatology, 5*(1), 25338. https://doi.org/10.3402/ejpt.v5.25338.

Tennen, H. & Affleck, G. (2005). Benefit-finding and benefit-reminding. In Snyder, C.R. & Lopez, S.J. (Eds.). *Handbook of Positive Psychology* (900pp. 584–597). Oxford University Press.

Thorgren, S., Wincent, J., & Sirén, C. (2013). The influence of passion and work–life thoughts on work satisfaction. *Human Resource Development Quarterly, 24*(4), 469–492. https://doi.org/10.1002/hrdq.21172.

Tonarelli, A., Cosenntino, C., Artioli, D., Borciani, S., Camurri, E., Colombo, B., D'Errico, A., Lelli, L., Lodini, L., & Artioli, G. (2017). Expressive writing. A tool to help health workers. Research project on the benefits of expressive writing. *Acta Biomed. 88*(5S), 13–21. https://doi.org/10.23750/abm.v88i5-S.6877

Vallerand, R. J., Blamchard, C., Mageau, G. A., Koestner, R., Ratelle, C., Léonard, M., & Gagné, M. (2003) Les Passions de l'Âme: On obsessive and harmonious passion. *J Pers Soc Psychol., 85*(4), 756–767. https://doi.org/10.1037/0022-3514.85.4.756

Vallerand, R. J., Paquet, Y., Philippe, F. L., & Charest, J. (2010). On the role of passion for work in burnout: A process model. *Journal of Personality, 78*(1), 289–312. https://doi.org/10.1111/j.1467-6494.2009.00616.x.

Zhang, N., Bai, B., & Zhu, J. (2023). Stress mindset, proactive coping behavior, and posttraumatic growth among health care professionals during the COVID-19 pandemic. *Psychological Trauma: Theory, Research, Practice, and Policy, 15*(3), 515–523. https://doi.org/10.1037/tra0001377.supp.

Zheng, X., Qu, J., & Xie, J., Yue, W., Liang, X., She, Z., Bai, J., Sun, Z., Cheng, F., Li, X., & Liu, C. (2022). Effectiveness of online expressive writing in reducing psychological distress among the asymptomatic COVID-19 patients in fangcang hospitals: A quasi-experiment study. *Frontiers in Psychology, 13*, 1042274. https://doi.org/10.3389/fpsyg.2022.1042274

Zhou, J. (2021). How does dualistic passion fuel academic thriving? A joint moderated-mediating model. *Frontiers in Psychology. 12*, 666830. https://doi.org/10.3389/fpsyg.2021.666830

8 Positive Psychology and Social Connection for Positive Health

Chapter Overview

This chapter provides an overview of the science of social connection and health and reviews applications of the PERMA model and other positive psychology strategies to increase high-quality, positive social connection. Social connection is associated with improved emotional, mental and physical health. Robust empirical evidence supports it as the key health factor for achieving positive health and increasing healthy longevity.

Introduction

"Other people matter" (Peterson, 2006) for our emotional, psychological, physiological and physical health. Social connection with family, friends, and community is a fundamental human need that has a significant impact on wellbeing. While empirical evidence of the link between social isolation and increased morbidity and mortality is strong (Holt-Lunstad et al., 2015), evidence for the inverse is also strong. Social connection is associated with a wide variety of health outcomes improvements, e.g. lower blood sugars, better cancer survival, decreased cardiovascular mortality, improved mental health, increased happiness, life satisfaction, and greater longevity (Holt-Lunstad et al., 2010, 2015; Martino et al., 2017;). Thus, care needs to be taken to help patients engage with others.

One of the best-known longitudinal studies, the Harvard Adult Development Study, which has been following study participants for over eight decades and is still ongoing corroborates other studies. When controlling for a wide range of confounders, the Harvard study found that the single most important factor in physical health, happiness, and longevity is social connection (Valliant, 2002; Waldinger & Schulz, 2022). Similarly, according to the decades of subjective wellbeing studies, positive relationships are the strongest predictors of wellbeing (Diener & Biswas-Diener, 2008). The good news is that despite its

DOI: 10.4324/9781003428909-8

links with personality and genetics, positive relationships are skills individuals can learn (Valliant, 2002), as such, it is important that physicians and the health care team consider it as part of the patient management plan.

By activating the parasympathetic nervous system and increasing vagal tone, positive social connection confers a number of physiologic benefits, including increased vagal tone. Moreover, the inverse has been shown; individuals with initially higher vagal tone levels increased their connectedness more rapidly than those with lower initial levels. Hence social connection and wellbeing can have a powerful reinforcing, reciprocal relationship (Kok & Fredrickson, 2010, 2016). Interestingly, although we often think of family and friends as our important social connections, when it comes to health and wellbeing, weak social ties, e.g. exchanges with acquaintances, can also contribute. A study found that on the days student participants interacted with more classmates than usual – they reported greater happiness and feelings of belonging (Sandstrom & Dunn, 2014). As such, all types of connections are important, close relationships, acquaintances as well as connections with strangers.

The reasons why social connection impacts our health and wellbeing are varied. For example, a longitudinal study has identified that happiness extends to three degrees of influence (Fowler & Christakis, 2008). Almost 5,000 people were followed over 20 years and clusters of happiness indicated that when a friend who lives nearby becomes happier, it increases our probability of happiness by 25%. A similar effect is observed in others from our circle of influence; the probability of our happiness increases by 8% when our spouse is happier, by 14% when our siblings are happier, and by 34% when our neighbors are happier. This means that social connections are not only good for us for the sake of it but can significantly impact our subjective wellbeing.

Also, according to the stress-buffering hypothesis (Cohen & Wills, 1985), when individuals who cope with daily stressors are supported by others, that support buffers the negative impact of the hassles and helps them cope more effectively with challenges. Partially, this could be due to experiencing higher levels of positive emotions when connecting with people. Those emotions then build psychological and emotional resources that help them cope with adversity and undo the negative effects of stressors, thus helping them experience less worry (Fredrickson, 2001).

Mechanisms of Action for Health in Positive Social Connections

During positive social connection, positive interpersonal processes can be enhanced by simultaneous genuine laughter, showing compassion and kindness, and shared positive experiences. These activities help to build high-quality social connections (Algoe, 2019; Kurtz & Algoe, 2017). For example, being kind increases the happiness of the giver; people are happier when they do good for others rather than themselves. Expressing gratitude to someone, not only increases the other's estimation of the grateful person and boosts their mood, but also improves the mood of the person expressing the gratitude (Algoe et al., 2016).

How a partner responds when something good happens is strongly related to the perception that the person will be there for them in the future during challenging times (Gable & Reis, 2010). In high-quality connections, both people sense mutual, positive regard, and share positive affect, mutual care and concern, resulting in behavioral and biological synchrony (Dutton & Heaphy, 2003; Major et al, 2018). The quality of one's interaction has a more significant effect on wellbeing than the quantity. Intentionally increasing quality can make up for the lower quantity.

Social connections help individuals endure, cope, become resilient, and potentially thrive in challenging times. Other benefits include buffering against depressive and illness symptoms. Quality social connections are associated with higher cognitive performance, faster recovery following loss and illness, higher levels of psychological safety, and greater collaboration (Lilius et al., 2008; Major et al, 2018; Stephens et al., 2013; Ybarra et al., 2008).

Positive Psychology Interventions (PPIs) for Social Connection

Positive emotions which are increased with PPIs, activities and mindsets can have a significant impact on positive social connection and psychological wellbeing, physical health, and cognitive function (Fredrickson, 2009). Positive affect enhances social relationships (Moore et al., 2018). Also, positive social connection boosts positive emotions; for example, research has reported that shared enjoyment influences positive affect (Arewasikporn et al., 2019). As with the other lifestyle medicine pillars, this reciprocal link can be leveraged in self-care and health care.

In previous chapters, we highlighted commonly studied PPIs that promote subjective and psychological wellbeing, including gratitude practice (Emmons & McCullough, 2003) and mindfulness (Keng et al., 2011). These interventions also contribute to improving social connections. In addition, identifying strengths, through the Virtues in Action (VIA) survey (https://www.viacharacter.org) and regularly using them in daily life is valuable for wellbeing. Strengths are positive qualities and attributes, such as kindness, creativity, and humor – which have been shown to boost wellbeing and life satisfaction and can positively impact social connections (Seligman, 2002).

In fact, when kindness and gratitude are practiced as self-focus or relationship-focused interventions, they result in different outcomes (O'Connell et al., 2016). In a self-focused group, participants were asked to praise themselves for something they have done and which they are grateful for; or, they were asked to do something kind to themselves and reflect on their feelings. Both these activities focused very much on individuals taking steps to make themselves happier. In a relationship-focused group, on the other hand, participants were asked to focus on others. They were asked to do something kind for someone in their network (friend, family, colleague) and reflect on how the receiver of their kindness felt; or they wrote and delivered an email, text, or face to face message to someone in their network, thanking them or praising them for something they were grateful for. The control group was asked to list three things that happened that day. When six weeks later, the results of all groups were compared with each other, the relationship-focused group reported the most significant improvements in wellbeing and relationship satisfaction. Most of the positive psychology and lifestyle medicine interventions are focused on individuals. Perhaps tweaking them to include the social aspect of an intervention can further maximize people's wellbeing.

Strengths can also serve as a way to connect with people. Identifying personal strengths can help individuals connect with others with similar strengths and values. Applying strengths, e.g. honesty, forgiveness, gratitude, leadership, and perseverance, to reach out to others in relationship-building ways can serve as an essential tool to support the critical social connection pillar of health and wellbeing (Niemiec & McGrath, 2019, viacharacter.org). Hence, partners who recognize and appreciate each others' strengths are more likely to feel satisfied with their relationship and feel they are growing (Kashdan et al., 2017).

Furthermore, specific strengths have been associated with developing and maintaining positive relationships. For example, curiosity promotes closeness in a relationship (Kashdan et al., 2011). Curious people expect more closeness with their partners and tend to feel closer to their partners during intimate chats. This is why, to develop such close relationships, it is essential to recognize each other's strengths and practice curiosity. Even if curiosity is not a top strengths, individuals may consider fostering curiosity for the sake of their relationships.

Character Strengths and Positive Relationships (Adapted from Veldorale-Brogan et al., 2010)

After completing a VIA character assessment, reflect on the new ways in which you can use your strengths to improve your relationships. For example, if one of your top strengths is kindness, consider what acts of kindness you could practice next week for your family, friends, colleagues, or strangers. If curiosity is one of your strengths, consider how you can rekindle your relationship with others by showing interest in them.

Over the years, psychology has focused a lot of attention on helping individuals figure out their relationship issues with their family and friends and find effective ways to resolve those issues as they improve and maintain their relationships. A positive psychology approach, however, also explores the positive aspects of communication, reasons why individuals became friends in the first place (Lyubomirksy & Layous, 2013), and how friends, family, and colleagues communicate in ways that keep their relationships positive. Reminiscence is a powerful tool for remembering and savoring relationships.

Positive Relationship Savoring (Adapted from Gander et al., 2016)

Reflect on three positive experiences with other people that happened today. Write them down and describe how you felt.

Research by Gable and colleagues (2010) showed that there are four distinct ways in which people react to each other's good news. We can either ignore the news, change the topic, become sarcastic about it, or completely disregard the excellent news. Alternatively, we can conditionally accept their good news, whereby we search for negatives in the good news. For example, a patient says they have started eating more fruit and vegetables over the last few weeks. Instead of praising them for it and celebrating their success, a physician may begin to point out that this is not enough and they need to introduce more healthy food into their diet. This type of approach will have a negative outcome on our relationship with the patient. The most constructive way to communicate is to allow the patient to feel proud and happy with the small changes they introduced. Praise them on those changes, celebrate them and only then, discuss how they can move it up a level. This approach, filled with appreciation, will lead to positive relationship development.

One more positive psychology technique that can promote social connectedness, positive emotions, and wellbeing is the practice of loving-kindness meditation, which involves directing positive emotions toward oneself and others (Fredrickson, 2013). Social support is another important factor in building connections and can be provided by family, friends, or even pets in the form of emotional support, advice, and assistance (Cohen & Wills, 1985). This kind of support buffers against the negative mental and physical effects of stress, serving a key role in a healthy lifestyle.

When discussing positive relations, we often consider friends, family, or colleagues from whom people give and receive support. However, positivity resonance theory suggests that we can benefit immensely from connecting with strangers (Fredrickson, 2016). They are the momentary connections that happen between people who know each other well or strangers, which are characterized by (1) shared positive affect, (2) mutual care and concern, and (3) behavioral and biological synchrony. For example, an elderly patient is sitting in a waiting room, and suddenly, her glasses fall off her nose onto the floor. A young patient, noticing it, jumps to his feet and helps pick up the glasses, and they both burst out laughing about the situation they share. In this moment, they may both experience positivity resonance. Experiencing this momentary positivity resonance is associated with psychological flourishing, reducing depression symptoms, loneliness, and illness symptoms (Major et al., 2018). Thus, creating positive resonance with patients can help them recover faster from illness and build a positive relationship with their physician and healthcare team.

Positive Psychology Approaches for High-Quality Social Connection

Several positive psychology tools can be applied in building positive social interactions. Listed below are examples of a few of these tools. Individuals can be encouraged to practice them as an investigatory exercise – evaluate how they feel afterward and decide how they may use them in work, school, family, and romantic relationships.

Positive reminiscence: After a positive experience interacting with someone, recall that experience and savor it; use that positive feeling to foster further positive connections.

Design a beautiful day: Write down or imagine a perfect day that involves positive social interactions. Envision the details of such a day, turn it into an action plan, and clear your schedule of other commitments for a day to make it come true.

Meaning: Reflect on the ways your relationships add meaning to your life. How do these people matter to you and how do you matter to them? Share your reflections with them.

Loving kindness meditation: Do a loving-kindness meditation for each of the important people in your life.

Positive self-portrait with social accomplishments: List ten ways you have been kind to others; list ten ways you have been lucky to meet and share life with family and friends; list ten ways you have been successful at creating positive relationships.

Strengths sharing: Make a date with a romantic partner, friend, or family member to share with each other the strengths you see in one another.

Strengths date: Make a date with a romantic partner and plan an activity that allows you to use as many of your top strengths as possible.

Clinical Applications of Positive Psychology for Social Connections

Health providers can apply principles of positive psychology in helping patients with social connections. They can also enhance how they implement lifestyle medicine competencies for this purpose.

Lifestyle Medicine Competencies: The Role of Connectedness and Positive Psychology

All of the lifestyle medicine competencies in the section on the role of connectedness and positive psychology are relevant to the topic of this book. Many of them can be expanded to promote social connection using its link with positive psychology approaches.

- When you apply positive psychology in health behavior change counseling, use these constructs to help patients build positive social connections.
- Describe how positive psychology strategies drive and support achieving and sustaining healthy behaviors; specifically describe how activities that boost positive emotions can leverage the upward spiral of lifestyle change, including behavior changes that build positive social connections.
- Describe how social connectedness and social networks affect emotional wellbeing, physical health, and longevity, including how positive interpersonal processes and positive emotions can improve social connections.
- Summarize the deleterious and positive effects social media has on emotional wellbeing and flourishing, including how authentic connections – via audio, virtual meetings, and in-person meetings – can boost positivity resonance; describe how positivity resonance is not usually experienced via social media.
- Explain the relationship among the lifestyle pillars, positive emotions, and flourishing, including how positive activities can serve as additional health protective factors at the core of positive health.
- Describe positive psychology activities that can boost emotional wellbeing and flourishing.

Table 8.1 shows the lifestyle medicine competencies for connectedness and positive psychology in the left column and recommends expansions of these competencies in a clinical practice that emphasizes social connection to facilitate positive health.

Table 8.1 Lifestyle medicine competencies: The role of connectedness and positive psychology

Lifestyle medicine competencies	Positive health expansion
Apply positive psychology in health behavior change counseling	Apply positive psychology constructs in helping patients make behavior changes that build positive social connections
Describe how positive psychology strategies support achieving and sustaining healthy behaviors	Describe how an initial focus on activities that boost positive emotions can leverage the upward spiral of lifestyle change, including behavior changes that support positive social connections
Describe how social connectedness and social networks affect emotional wellbeing, physical health, and longevity	Describe how positive interpersonal processes and positive emotions can improve social connections, leading to greater wellbeing benefits
Summarize the deleterious and positive effects social media has on emotional wellbeing and flourishing	Summarize how authentic connections, via phone, virtual meetings, and in-person meetings, can boost positivity resonance – which is not usually experienced via social media
Explain the relationship among the lifestyle pillars, positive emotions, and flourishing	Explain how positive activities, especially positive social interaction, boost positive emotions and serve as additional health protective factors independent of traditional risk factors; describe how when combined with the healthy lifestyle pillars, represent the core of flourishing and positive health
Describe positive psychology activities that can boost emotional wellbeing and flourishing	Describe how positive activities not only promote emotional wellbeing but also lay the foundation of flourishing, along with other healthy lifestyle pillars, in the emerging field of positive health

Application of PERMA in the Context of Positive Social Connections

In the outline below suggest questions based on the PERMA framework that the health provider or other team members can pose to patients for driving positive social connections.

P—Positive emotions: Engage in activities that increase positive feelings and build positive social connections.
- What kinds of activities give you positive feelings, especially when around others?

- How can you best pay attention to positive experiences when you are spending time with family and friends?

E—Engagement (Flow): Engage in activities that get you fully immersed while sharing them with others, such as playing musical instruments or dancing together.
- What activities that involve others have given you a sense of flow?
- What new activities that involve others and produce a sense of flow would you like to try?

R—Relationships: Identify how you can increase positive social interactions and improve social connections.
- What enjoyable social activities can you increase?
- Who can you connect with positively?
- How can you improve your social connections?

M—Meaning: Pay attention to the social activities in your life that feel meaningful.
- What are meaningful activities you can do with others?
- How can you take action to increase social connections that give you a sense of meaning and life purpose?
- How have you supported others in ways that feel meaningful?

A—Achievement: Celebrate progress toward positive social connectivity goals.
- What social activities have you engaged in that make you feel proud?
- How have you supported others in ways that are fulfilling and give you a sense of accomplishment?

Appreciative Inquiry to Increase Positive Social Connections

Just as with other pillars, an appreciative inquiry process can help support individuals in taking actions that engage in positive social interactions and build high-quality connections.

Discovery: What is good now?
- What habits do you maintain that help you connect positively with others?
- How do you positively interact with people you do not know well during the course of the day, e.g. authentic greetings?
- What enjoyable activities do you engage in with others?
- Which personal strengths have been important in making and maintaining healthy relationships?

Dream: What changes are possible to improve positive social interactions and increase connections?
- What changes are possible for building high-quality connections?
- What would a life with greater social connections look like?

Design: What positive changes could you make to build social connections?
- What new social activities could you engage in?
- What favorite positive activity could you do with others?
- How can you use your personal strengths to build high-quality connections?

Destiny: What changes to build social connections are you confident and ready you can make?
- What action plan are you ready to make for increasing and improving your social connections?
- Which personal strengths will you use to engage in positive interactions?
- What are healthy ways to reward yourself as you achieve your action plan?

Practice Tools: Social Connection Prescription and Action Plan Example

Social connection can be included in a prescription as with other healthy lifestyle pillars. An example follows:

Social Connection Prescription

Connect in person or via phone with a friend or family member three times every week.

Use the three S's for support:

Sharing: Ask a friend or family member to check on your progress.
Strengths: Use your top strengths to meet your goal, such as kindness to connect and help others.
Savoring: Savor the good feelings during and after your social interactions.

Refills: Unlimited

Perspectives on Practicing from the Inside Out – Social Connection

Positive interactions with co-workers and with patients throughout a busy workday can serve the health practitioner, their coworkers, and the patients well. Intentionally building micro-moments of positivity resonance will build and support everyone's wellbeing. This process that is witnessed by the patient during the clinical encounter can become a memorable role model to be adapted outside of the health care settings. Moments of authentic sharing and listening, shared laughter and kindness can go a long way.

Many positive psychology-based activities and principles can be harnessed for this purpose, such as keeping a gratitude jar in the clinic, where workers drop in notes of gratitude throughout the week, and these notes are read during team huddles. This activity can bring the team closer together. When each team member sets a goal to do a series of kind acts over a few days, their health will benefit and they will build pro-social behaviors and high-quality connections that support the team during demanding and stressful times (Gherghel et al, 2019; Hui et al., 2020). Also, kind acts to patients are shown to improve patients' subjective perception of care (Hake & Post, 2023).

As we've seen, the most robust cohort studies, confirm the power of social connection for our health and wellbeing. Even if a clinical practice does not have the capacity to make any other changes, intentionally planning as a group and making these changes to maximize positive interaction is the single, most important place to start.

Case Study of Positive Health Clinical Approaches for Social Connection

Patient Background: Ed is a 56-year-old engineer of Asian descent with hypertension who was diagnosed with major depressive disorder six months ago. He has a history of chronic stress due to work and family demands, and he has been experiencing symptoms of depression such as persistent sadness, loss of interest in activities, decreased energy, and insomnia, but denies thoughts of suicide. He chose your practice after a change in his health insurance coverage. His previous physician prescribed antidepressant medication, a selective serotonin reuptake inhibitor, and psychotherapy. Ed has been taking the medication, but he is not interested in psychotherapy. His symptoms have not improved significantly after two months of taking the medication.

Assessment: Screening with Patient Health Questionnaire 9 (PHQ 9) results in a score of 15 and diagnostic evaluation with the Hamilton Rating Scale for Depression (HAM-D) produces a score of 17, indicating moderate depression.

Treatment Plan: The health team, consisting of his primary care provider and social worker, recommends that action steps to promote social connection be included in his treatment plan. They believe that Mr. John's lack of social support and isolation contributed to his depression and that improving his social connections could enhance his mental health. The social worker conducts a social assessment and identifies that Mr. John has a limited social network due to his busy work schedule and family responsibilities. He has no close friends and does not participate in social activities outside of work. The social worker discusses with Mr. John the benefits of social connection on mental health and suggests strategies to increase his social connections.

Intervention: The treatment team develops a social connection intervention plan for Mr. John, which includes the following:

1   Social skills training: The social worker provides Mr. John with social skills training to enhance his communication and interpersonal skills. The training includes active listening, expressing emotions effectively, and building rapport.
2   Social activity planning: The social worker and Mr. John identify social activities that he can participate in regularly. They also identify a local community center that offers a range of activities, such as group exercise classes, art classes, and support groups.
3   Volunteer work: The social worker suggests that Mr. John volunteers for a local charity organization. This activity can, not only provide him with an opportunity to contribute to the community but also help him meet new people.
4   Support group: The social worker identifies a local support group for individuals with depression. Mr. John agreed to attend the group and participate in weekly meetings.

Outcome: After three months of the social connection intervention, Mr. John shows improvement in his depression symptoms. He reports feeling less sad and more energized. He also reports that he has made a new friend and has participated in several social activities, which he enjoyed. His follow-up HAM-D score is 10. The social worker conducts a follow-up social assessment and notes that Mr. John's social network has expanded, and he has become more socially engaged.

Key Take-Aways: The case of Mr. John demonstrates the importance of social connection as part of depression treatment. Incorporating social connection interventions, such as social skills training, social activity planning, volunteer work, and support groups – can enhance mental and physical health outcomes. Hence, social connection interventions should be considered as a standard part of a comprehensive lifestyle-oriented treatment plan for achieving positive health.

Conclusion

Social connection is a fundamental human need that has a significant impact on wellbeing. Positive psychology techniques, including loving-kindness meditation and social support, can be effective in promoting social connection and improving wellbeing. Positive interpersonal processes, such as shared laughter and compassion and expressions of gratitude for one another, can be applied in various settings, including healthcare settings, to help individuals become physically healthier, happier, and lead longer and more fulfilling lives. A lifestyle medicine practice that is oriented to facilitating positive health can assess the social networks of its patients and implement interventions based on the PERMA, appreciative inquiry, action plans supported by the three S's – sharing, strengths, and savoring – to promote the social connection pillar. Moreover, positive interactions between providers and patients and among health team members serve as role models for the patients, as well as lead to positivity resonance with mental, emotional, and physical benefits for both the patients and the health care team.

References

Algoe, S. B. (2019). Positive interpersonal processes. *Current Directions in Psychological Science*, *28*(2), 183–188. https://doi.org/10.1177/0963721419827272.

Algoe, S. B., Kurts, L. E., & Hlaire, N. M. (2016). Putting the you in "thank you": Examining other praising behavior as the active relational component in expressed gratitude. *Social Psychological and Personality Science*, *7*(3), 658–666. https://doi.org/10.1177/1948550616651681.

Arewasikporn, A., Sturgein, J. A., & Zautra, A. J. (2019). Sharing positive experiences boosts resilient thinking: Everyday benefits of social connection and positive emotion in a community sample. *American Journal of Community Psychology*, *63*(1–2), 110–121. https://doi.org/10.1002/ajcp.12279.

Cohen, S., & Wills, T. A. (1985). Stress, social support, and the buffering hypothesis. *Psychological Bulletin*, *98*(2), 310–357.

Diener, E., & Biswas-Diener, R. (2008). *Happiness: Unlocking the mysteries of psychological wealth*. Blackwell Publishing. https://doi.org/10.1002/9781444305159

Dutton, J. E., & Heaphy, E. D. (2003). The power of high functioning connections. In K. Cameron, & J. Dutton (Eds.), *Positive organizational scholarship: Foundations of a new discipline* (pp. 212–278). Berret-Koehler Publishers.

Emmons, R. A., & McCullough, M. E. (2003). Counting blessings versus burdens: An experimental investigation of gratitude and subjective well-being in daily life. *Journal of Personality and Social Psychology*, *84*(2), 377–389. https://doi.org/10.1037/0022-3514.84.2.377.

Fowler, J. H., & Christakis, N. A. (2008). Dynamic spread of happiness in a large social network: Longitudinal analysis over 20 years in the Framingham heart study. *BMJ (Clinical Research Ed.)*, *337*, a2338. https://doi.org/10.1136/bmj.a2338

Fredrickson, B. L. (2001). The role of positive emotions in positive psychology: The broaden-and-build theory of positive emotions. *American Psychologist*, *56*(3), 218–226. https://doi.org/10.1037/0003-066X.56.3.218.

Fredrickson, B. L. (2009). *Positivity.* Crown Publishers.

Fredrickson, B. L. (2013). Positive emotions broaden and build. In S. J. Lopez & C. R. Snyder (Eds.), *Oxford handbook of positive psychology* (2nd ed., pp. 129–143). Oxford University Press.

Fredrickson, B. L. (2016). Love: Positivity resonance as a fresh, evidence-based perspective on an age-old topic. In L.F. Barrett & J.M. Haviland (Eds.), *Handbook of emotions* (4th ed., pp. 847–858). Guilford Press.

Gable, S. L., & Reis, H. (2010). Good news! Capitalizing on positive events in an interpersonal context. *Advances in Experimental Social Psychology, 42,* 195–257. https://doi.org/10.1016/S0065-2601(10)42004-3

Gander, F., Proyer, R. T., & Ruch, W. (2016). Positive psychology interventions addressing pleasure, engagement, meaning, positive relationships, and accomplishment increase well-being and ameliorate depressive symptoms: A randomized, placebo-controlled online study. *Frontiers in Psychology, 7,* 686. https://doi.org/10.3389/fpsyg.2016.00686

Hake, A. B., & Post, S. G. (2023). Kindness: Definitions and a pilot study for the development of a kindness scale in healthcare. *PLoS One, 18*(7), e0288766. https://doi.org/10.1371/journal.pone.0288766.

Holt-Lunstad, J., Smith, T. B., & Baker, M., Harris, T., & Stephenson, D. (2015). Loneliness and social isolation as risk factors for mortality: A meta-analytic review. *Perspectives on Psychological Science, 10*(2), 227–237. https://doi.org/10.1177/1745691614568352

Holt-Lunstad, J., Smith, T. B., & Layton, J. B. (2010). Social relationships and mortality risk: A meta-analytic review. *PLoS Medicine, 7*(7). https://doi.org/10.1371/journal.pmed.1000316

Hui, B. P. H., Ng, J. C. K., Berzaghi, E., Cunningham-Amos, L. A., & Kogan, A. (2020). Rewards of kindness? A meta-analysis of the link between prosociality and well-being. *Psychological Bulletin, 146*(12), 1084–1116.

Kashdan, T. B., McKnight, P. E., Fincham, F. D., & Rose, P. (2011). When curiosity breeds intimacy: Taking advantage of intimacy opportunities and transforming boring conversations. *Journal of Personality, 79,* 1369–1401. https://doi.org/10.1111/j.1467-6494.2010.00697.x

Keng, S. L., Smoski, M. J., & Robins, C. J. (2011). Effects of mindfulness on psychological health: A review of empirical studies. *Clinical Psychology Review, 31*(6), 1041–1056. https://doi.org/10.1016/j.cpr.2011.04.006.

Kok, B. E., & Fredrickson, B. L. (2010). Upward spirals of the heart: Autonomic flexibility, as indexed by vagal tone, reciprocally and prospectively predicts positive emotions and social connectedness. *Biological Psychology, 85,* 432–436. https://doi.org/10.1016/j.biopsycho.2010.09.005

Kok, B. E., & Fredrickson, B. L. (2016). Corrigendum to "upward spirals of the heart: Autonomic flexibility, as indexed by vagal tone, reciprocally and prospectively predicts positive emotions and social connectedness" [Biol. Psychol. 85 (3) (2010) 432–436]. *Biological Psychology, 117,* 240. https://doi.org/10.1016/j.biopsycho.2016.03.001

Kurtz, L. E., & Algoe, S. B. (2017). When sharing a laugh means sharing more: Testing the role of shared laughter on short-term interpersonal consequences. Journal of Nonverbal Behavior, 41, 34–65. https://doi.org/10.1007/s10919-016-0245-9

Lilius, J. M., Worline, M. C., Maitlis, S., Kanov, J., Dutton, J. E., & Frost, P. (2008). The contours and consequences of compassion at work. *Journal of Organizational Behavior, 29,* 193–218. https://doi.org/10.1002/job.508

Lyubomirsky, S., & Layous, K. (2013). How do simple positive activities increase wellbeing? *Curr Dir Psychol Sci.*, *22*(1), 57–62. https://doi.org/10.1177/0963721412469809

Major, B. C., Le Nguyen, K. D., Lundberg, K. B., & Fredrickson, B. L. (2018). Wellbeing correlates of perceived positivity resonance: Evidence from trait and episode-level assessments. *Personality and Social Psychology Bulletin, 44*(12), 1631–1647. https://doi.org/10.1177/0146167218771324

Martino, J., Pegg, J., & Frates, E. P. (2017). The connection prescription: Using the power of social interactions and the deep desire for connectedness to empower health and wellness. *American Journal of Lifestyle Medicine, 11*(6), 466–475. https://doi.org/10.1177/1559827615608788.

Moore, S. M., Diener, E., & Tan, K. (2018). Using multiple methods to more fully understand causal relations: Positive affect enhances social relationships. In E. Diener, S. Oshi, & L. Tay (Eds.), *Handbook of wellbeing* (pp. 1–17). DEF Publishers.

Niemiec, R., & McGrath, R. E. (2019). *The power of character strengths, an official guide from the VIA Institute on Character.* VIA Institute on Character.

O'Connell, B. H., O'Shea, D., & Gallagher, S. (2016). Enhancing social relationships through positive psychology activities: A randomised controlled trial. *The Journal of Positive Psychology, 11*(2), 149–162. https://doi.org/10.1080/17439760.2015.1037860.

Peterson, C. (2006). *A primer in positive psychology.* Oxford University Press.

Sandstrom, G., & Dunn, E. (2014). Social interactions and well-being: The surprising power of weak ties. *Personality and Social Psychology Bulletin, 40*, 910–922.

Seligman, M. E. P. (2002). *Authentic happiness: Using the new positive psychology to realize your potential for lasting fulfillment.* Free Press.

Stephens, J. P., Heaphy, E. D., Carmel, A., Spreitzer, G. M., & Dutton, J. E. (2013). Relationship quality and virtuousness: Emotional carrying capacity as a source of individual and team resilience. *The Journal of Applied Behavioral Science, 49*(1), 13–41. https://doi.org/10.1177/0021886312471193

Valliant, G. E. (2002). *Aging well: Surprising guideposts to a happier life from the landmark Harvard study of adult development.* Little Brown.

Veldorale-Brogan, A., Bradford, K., & Vail, A. (2010). Marital virtues and their relationship to individual functioning, communication, and relationship adjustment. *The Journal of Positive Psychology, 5*(4), 281–293. https://doi.org/10.1080/17439760.2010.498617.

Ybarra, O., Burnstein, E., Winkelman, P. Keller, M. C., Manis, M, Chan, E., & Rodriguez, J. (2008). Mental exercising through simple socializing: Social interaction promotes general cognitive functioning. *Personality and Social Psychology Bulletin, 34*(2), 248–259. d https://doi.org/10.1177/0146167207310454

Waldinger, R., & Schulz, M. (2022). *The good life.* Simon & Schuster.

9 Positive Health for Patients with Chronic Medical Conditions

Chapter Overview

This chapter provides a brief review of the scientific study of the association of positive psychology constructs in the context of chronic diseases and medical conditions, including cardiovascular disease, diabetes, arthritis, and asthma. The scientific literature about the impact of positive psychology interventions (PPIs) on the outcomes of these diseases is also highlighted. Applications of positive psychology and more broadly, positive health – which combine healthy living, positive psychology, and other factors in the biopsychosocial model – in health care can not only improve the health of individuals with common chronic, lifestyle-related, diseases mediated through biological, behavioral, and psychosocial pathways but also lead to flourishing despite these conditions.

Introduction

According to the World Health Organization, chronic diseases, including cancer, heart disease, stroke, and diabetes – are responsible for approximately 74% of all deaths worldwide (World Health Organization, 2022). In addition, these conditions are major contributors to poor mental and emotional health, disability, lost productivity, and reduced quality of life (Benkel et al., 2020; Hajat & Stein, 2018; Maresova et al., 2019). Since 1990, the burden from chronic diseases and injuries has significantly shifted to represent the greatest proportion of years lost due to disability (GBD 2019 Diseases and Injuries Collaborators, 2020).

Chronic diseases often have significant impacts on an individual's emotional wellbeing, resulting in anxiety, depression, and stress. For example, individuals with cancer may experience fear of recurrence, while those with diabetes may worry about the potential for complications. Such emotions can have negative

DOI: 10.4324/9781003428909-9

effects on an individual's physical and psychological health, including impaired immune function and increased risk of cardiovascular disease.

Therefore, chronic diseases can require significant resources and support from healthcare professionals, family, and friends. Traditional medical treatments often focus on symptom management, disease control, and prevention of complications. These treatments do not address the underlying cause of the diseases, nor do they fully address the emotional and psychological impact of chronic diseases on individuals. A comprehensive healthy lifestyle – with a plant-predominant eating pattern, physical activity, restorative sleep, reducing risky substance use, and social connection along with mindsets and activities based on positive psychology that reduce stress and increase positive emotions – offers a more powerful approach. This positive health clinical practice drives prevention and treatment of the underlying pathophysiologic mechanisms at the root of chronic diseases and promotes all major elements of health – mental, emotional, physical, social, and spiritual – leading to positive health.

The Role of Positive Psychology in Improving Health for Patients with Chronic Diseases

Positive psychology aims to promote positive emotions, behaviors, and thoughts and focus on an individual's strengths and abilities rather than their weaknesses and limitations. When included in comprehensive lifestyle treatment, positive psychology activities offer a promising approach to, not only complement and enhance, but also revolutionize traditional medical treatments for chronic diseases. This approach can lead to physical, mental and emotional health, as well as effective coping, resilience, thriving, and even growth in the face of medical disease and other adversities.

The empirical literature suggests a prospective association between positive psychological states, such as positive emotions, life satisfaction, optimism, life purpose and social support, and good physical health. Subjective wellbeing that can be improved through positive psychology interventions (PPIs) as shown in scientific reviews (Hendriks et al., 2020) has been closely linked to physical health (Cross et al., 2018) with positive impact on short and long-term health outcomes, such as immune response (Howell et al, 2007). Also, higher purpose has been associated with better health in mid and later years of life (Willroth et al., 2021).

PPIs that can lead to positive emotions include proactive intentional activities for wellbeing. Examples include gratitude journaling about positive aspects of one's life, mindfulness with a focus on the present moment, and positive reappraisal that involves re-evaluating negative experiences in a more positive light, which can help individuals struggling with chronic diseases. These interventions cultivate positive emotions, for example, joy and hope. PPIs have also been found to be effective in reducing symptoms of depression and anxiety in individuals with various chronic conditions, including cancer, heart disease, and diabetes – hence improving both emotional and mental health (Segerstrom & Sephton, 2010; Emmons & McCullough, 2003; Huffman et al., 2011).

A systemic review and meta-analysis of eight randomized, controlled outcomes studies of mindfulness-based stress reduction (MBSR) found small, but significant effects on lowering depression, anxiety, and psychological distress (Bohlmeijer et al., 2010). Moreover, a meta-analysis of 30 randomized, controlled trials that studied PPIs among 1,864 adult participants with psychiatric (primarily depressive and anxiety disorders) or somatic disorders (primarily cancer, cardiac disease) points to mental and physical improvement. The PPIs, including gratitude, kindness, and meaning-making interventions, showed a small, but significant effect on wellbeing and depression and a moderate effect on anxiety. The researchers concluded that PPIs should be considered for patients with somatic disorders, as well as patients with diseases that are primarily psychological in nature (Chakhssi et al., 2018).

Spotlight on Positive Psychology's Role in Physical Health

Most of us are likely not to be surprised that positive psychology is associated with subjective wellbeing and emotional and mental health, but the link with physical health may not be as intuitive. Yet, as we highlighted, positive psychology can impact physical health along with other elements of health.

One mechanism for positive psychology's role in physical health suggested by scientific studies is the positive impact of subjective wellbeing – boosted by positive emotions – on physical health. In a general population study, subjective wellbeing, positive feelings, and global life satisfaction significantly predicted lowered risks of all-cause and natural and unnatural-cause mortality, after controlling for major confounding variables (Xu & Roberts, 2010).

Ed Diener, a leading and highly cited positive psychology researcher, concluded that high subjective wellbeing, especially life satisfaction, optimism, and positive emotions, leads to improved physical health and longevity, even when controlling for baseline health and socioeconomic status (Diener & Chan, 2011). An important question highly relevant to health care and self-care is whether intentional, proactive PPIs can improve physical health outcomes. More research is especially needed to study outcomes of PPIs as part of treatment in medical settings.

While that research is ongoing, incorporating PPIs into a comprehensive healthy lifestyle may be prudent. We can design positive health approaches based on the logic model that pulls together existing studies, showing how PPIs boost positive emotions and, in turn, positive emotions are associated with various elements of health. This logic model weaves in several underlying mechanisms of action for positive emotions, some of which are increased by PPIs. Positive emotions as referred to here include, not only hedonic ones such as joy and pleasant feelings, but also optimism, hope and eudaimonic

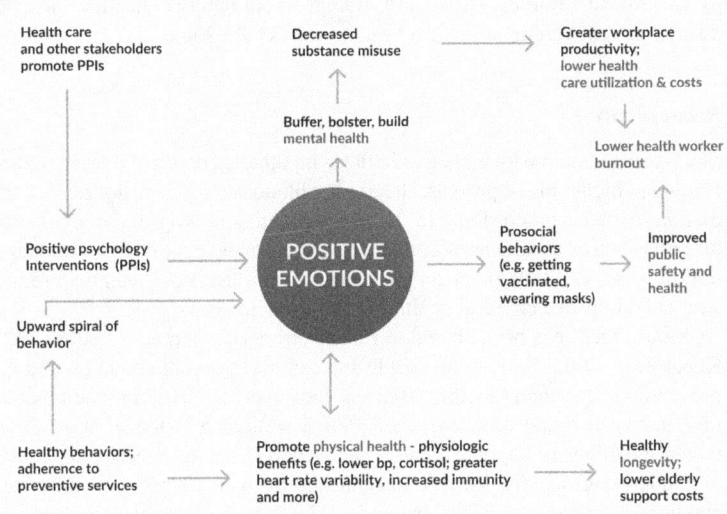

Figure 9.1 How are positive emotions connected with different elements of health – combined to achieve positive health? (Copyright permission granted by the Global Positive Health Institute).

emotions that arise from meaningful activities. As shown in Figure 9.1, these positive emotions are linked with better health, quality of life, and longevity with benefits to individuals, health systems and societies.

Underlying Mechanisms of Action of PPIs for Positive Health

While there is still much to be learned about the relationship between positive psychology and physical health, research suggests several underlying mechanisms for the impact of PPIs via biological, behavioral, and psychosocial pathways.

Healthy Behaviors

One specific mechanism of action of positive psychology relevant to lifestyle medicine is the power of positive emotions to nonconsciously drive healthy behaviors (Van Cappellen et al., 2017), such as healthy eating and physical activity, that counter underlying inflammatory and pathologic processes common to a wide spectrum of diseases. This process that leverages positive emotions can advance the outcomes of behavior change techniques, such as self-efficacy training, skills, and strategies – to facilitate healthy lifestyles needed to treat chronic diseases (Luszczynska et al., 2009).

Reduced Stress

Stress is associated with increases in the sympathetic nervous system response leading to higher blood pressure, heart rate, blood sugars, cortisol, and inflammation, which can contribute to the development and progression of chronic diseases such as cardiovascular disease, diabetes, and cancer. PPIs, including mindfulness, gratitude practice, and positive reminiscence – can help reduce stress and improve physical health via these mechanisms.

Mindfulness has been shown to reduce stress (Bartlett et al., 2019, 2021; Kabat-Zinn, 2003; Keng et al., 2011) and can decrease inflammation and improve immune system function (Black & Savich et al., 2016). Practicing gratitude has been found to improve subjective wellbeing (Alkozei et al, 2018) increase feelings of happiness and reduce stress (Sansone & Sansone, 2010).

Underlying negative health mechanisms by which stress and other risk conditions operate, especially the activated sympathetic nervous system and increased inflammation, may be countered by positive psychological physiologic benefits. The ways in which positive psychology and positive health approaches benefit individuals with medical conditions are introduced below.

Decreased Inflammatory Processes and Improved Immune System

Detrimental inflammatory processes may be countered by positive psychology physiologic processes independently of driving healthy behaviors. For example, experiencing awe has been shown to be a strong predictor of lower proinflammatory cytokine levels, after controlling for different personality and health variables (Stellar et al., 2015). Also, gratitude has been associated with lower inflammatory markers in asymptomatic heart failure patients (Mills et al., 2015). Positive emotions, such as happiness and optimism, have been linked to improved immune system function (Pressman & Black, 2012). However, more research is needed to validate the effect of specific PPIs, such as practicing gratitude or engaging in acts of kindness, on the immune system function.

Increased Use of Personal Strengths

The positive psychology approach which emphasizes personal strengths gives individuals a sense of agency over their lives and can build capacity to thrive despite difficulties, such as those presented by medical illness. For example, solution-focused therapy, which involves focusing on an individual's strengths and resources rather than their problems and limitations and setting proactive goals has been found to be effective in improving wellbeing, reducing symptoms of depression and anxiety and improving self-efficacy important in health behaviors and quality of life in individuals with chronic conditions, including cancer, heart disease, and diabetes (Xu & Roberts, 2010; Zhang et al., 2018).

Greater and More Effective Social Support

Positive health practice which emphasizes the role of social connection can help people with chronic diseases by promoting social support. Social support is essential for managing chronic diseases, as it can help people feel less isolated and provide practical assistance with daily tasks. PPIs, such as expressing gratitude and engaging in acts of kindness, can help strengthen social connections and promote social support (Liao & Weng, 2018; Smith 2018).

For example, a study of an intervention that involved expressing gratitude to loved ones helped people with heart failure feel more socially connected and improved their overall wellbeing. The 70 participants with heart failure were randomly assigned to either the intervention – writing letters that expressed gratitude to loved ones – or a control group. The participants in the gratitude group reported significant improvements in social connectedness and overall wellbeing compared to the control group (Redwine et al., 2016).

Also, social support in the form of seeking and receiving emotional, informational, and practical support from others has been found to promote healthy behaviors, such as increased physical activity, in individuals with cancer, heart disease, diabetes, and other chronic diseases (DiMatteo, 2004).

Self-compassion

Practicing self-compassion, that is being kind and understanding toward oneself in the face of difficulties or failures, is another positive psychology approach that can support physical health. This practice can improve emotional wellbeing but also has been found to be effective in promoting healthy behaviors, including increased physical activity and better nutrition, in individuals with chronic diseases, such as diabetes and heart disease (Sirois et al., 2015).

Achieving Positive Health in Patient Populations

The combined powerful approach of addressing traditional risk factors, as well as increasing health protective factors through positive psychology, along with other elements of the biopsychosocial model, including environmental supports, can lead to a state of positive health. A common definition of positive health is still under development. Positive health is seen by some leaders in the field as both a journey and a destination of health. It is spurred and propagated by healthy lifestyles and positive psychology-based habits aiming for less frequent, briefer ailments, greater ability to recuperate, rapid wound healing, more physiological reserves, chronic diseases that are less debilitating (Park et al., 2014) and greater happiness, life satisfaction and longevity (Diener & Chan, 2011).

Although more research is needed, current research points to small, but significant effects of PPIs on individual positive health and wellbeing. The PPIs may have more significant effects when offered to patient populations and the community more broadly. As chronic diseases are the most common conditions across developed and developing countries and patients with chronic diseases are cared for by lifestyle medicine, primary care, and many other medical specialties – designing health care in these settings to offer medical services that prioritize positive health has significant potential to improve the overall health of populations. Progress of health care toward achieving positive health can be measured in multiple ways. For example, early adopters have proposed using the measure of happiness-adjusted life expectancies (HLEs) – the product of the average life expectancy and the average happiness, as assessed by measures such as subjective wellbeing and life satisfaction (Veenhoven, 1996).

Positive Psychology for Specific Medical Conditions

This section highlights scientific studies of positive psychology applications for patients with several specific common chronic diseases: cardiovascular disease, diabetes, arthritis, and asthma.

Cardiovascular Disease

One disease category that is commonly treated in lifestyle medicine and primary care practices is cardiovascular disease. Empirical studies suggest a robust association between positive emotions and cardiovascular disease outcomes (Sin et al, 2017). Ten prospective studies with 136,265 participants found a 17% decrease in all-cause mortality and a 17% decrease in cardiovascular events for those with a higher purpose in life (Cohen et al., 2016). Researchers corroborated this significant finding for cardiovascular disease (CVD) (Kim et al., 2013a) and stroke (Kim et al., 2013b). An example of a specific positive psychology construct prospectively associated with cardiovascular health is optimism (Kubzansky et al., 2018).

Moreover, the findings of a study group in the National Health and Nutrition Examination Survey I 6,025 US men and women aged from 25 to 74 years without coronary heart disease at baseline – followed for a mean of 15 years reported that high baseline levels of emotional vitality were associated with an adjusted relative risk 19% lower than those with low emotional vitality. Even after controlling for health behaviors and other potential confounders, including depressive symptoms, a significant dose-response relationship was reported (Kubzansky & Thurston, 2007).

Other studies corroborate this association between positive psychology constructs, lower cardiovascular disease rates, and better outcomes (Boehm et al., 2011, 2021; Boehm & Kubzansky, 2012; Dubois et al., 2015; Masters et al., 2020). It's also no surprise that associations between CVD risk factors and positive psychology-based activities have been shown, such as the prospective association of volunteerism with a lower risk of hypertension. In the latter study, the volunteer group also experienced better psychological wellbeing and greater physical activity, but in the analyzes, these factors did not explain the lower blood pressure levels (Sneed & Cohen, 2013).

The association between positive psychology constructs and CVD is complex and needs further research to tease out key factors that could be applied clinically. In one study, life satisfaction was associated with lower cardiometabolic risk scores, but positive emotions were not. One explanation could be that life satisfaction may correlate with meaningful activities and life purpose – which have been shown to impact physical health (Kim et al., 2022) – rather than purely pleasurable ones. This suggests that PPIs that are multi-modal and address a range of positive psychology constructs may be prudent, while the research identifies the most impactful factors.

A key question for a clinical practice focused on increasing positive health is whether intentionally implementing PPIs can improve CVD outcomes. PPIs have been shown to improve psychological wellbeing in patients. For example, in a group of post-cardiac procedure patients who were randomized to receive PPIs or wait-listed, although no differences in wellbeing were noted post-interventions, depression was decreased and happiness and hope increased significantly for the intervention group at follow-up (Nikrahan et al., 2016). In turn psychological wellbeing, has been associated with cardiovascular health and other health elements. Major mechanisms of action may include health behavior change support, stress reduction, psychosocial support, and improvements in protective physiologic factors, such as lowered blood pressure. Therefore, although initial studies show mixed results on specific risk factors, such as blood pressure, when considering the impact of PPIs on health behavior, stress and social connection, positive psychology assessments and interventions in the context of CVD treatment have been recommended (Gaffey et al., 2024; Kubzansky et al., 2018; Levine et al., 2021). Moreover, PPIs have been shown to be feasible and well-accepted in cardiac care settings. (Petersen et al., 2016; Hernandez et al., 2018; Huffman et al., 2011; Sin, 2016). However rigorous intervention trials to study outcomes are needed.

Diabetes

The association with and impact of positive psychology constructs and practices on the development and outcomes of diabetes have also been studied. As with CVD and other medical conditions, further research is needed; early studies support including positive activities in diabetes care.

Associations have been found between positive wellbeing and resilience and quality of life of patients with Type 1 diabetes (Yi-Frazier et al., 2015). For example, in one study PPIs increased quality of life and happiness for patients with Type 2 diabetes (Assarzadegan & Raeisi, 2019). For both Types 1 and 2 diabetes, positive personal characteristics, such as self-efficacy and positive environmental factors and support – are associated with better management and outcomes of the disease (Yi-Frazier et al., 2012). Also, positive affect is linked with lower mortality from diabetes (Moskowitz et al., 2008). In terms of prevention, life satisfaction and emotional vitality have been associated with a lower risk of a diagnosis of diabetes (Boehm et al., 2015).

Feasible healthcare designs for integrating PPIs into care have been developed (Dubois et al., 2016; Jasper et al., 2020), and glycemic control results after PPI programs compared to traditional diabetes education programs are being studied (Jasper et al., 2020). Early intervention trials support using positive psychology-based exercises with motivational interviewing approaches for improved health behavior adherence and modest benefits on body mass index and hemoglobin A1c (Celano et al., 2018).

Specifically, having a sense of meaning and purpose may be a key factor in diabetes care and other chronic diseases. Authors of a study of purpose and healthy behaviors recommend interventions that target this positive psychology construct to help older adults maintain some healthy behaviors (Kim et al., 2020). Driving and supporting health behaviors is an important mechanism for better medical outcomes for patients with diabetes, including glycemic control and lower mortality rates (Massey et al., 2017). For example, incorporating positive psychology into motivational interviewing has been effective in promoting a key behavior in the management of diabetes, namely physical activity (Zambrano et al., 2020; Huffman et al., 2021).

Arthritis

Another chronic illness that may be impacted by positive psychology constructs is arthritis. Perceived social support, hope, optimism, and resilience may serve as effective alleviators of the fatigue that often is experienced by patients with rheumatoid arthritis, with the first of these showing the greatest effect (Xu et al., 2017). In addition, studies suggest that optimism, benefit finding, gratitude, and self-compassion can help patients with adjusting to this illness (Sirois, 2014).

Gratitude was also shown in a longitudinal study to be a significant predictor of thriving and lower depression, among patients with arthritis, as well as those with inflammatory bowel disease (Sirois & Wood, 2017). In addition, empirical data suggest that positive psychology strategies, such as self-compassionate acceptance, optimism, adaptive coping, and family and social support may improve the efficacy of arthritis treatments, possibly through changes in the neuro-endocrine-immune pathways (Santiago et al., 2015).

Early studies of proactive PPIs for arthritis management show promise. For example, in one study of an online mindfulness and gratitude intervention, pain anxiety, pain intensity, fear of movement, and pain self-efficacy were improved (Swain et al., 2020).

Asthma

Patients with asthma may benefit from PPIs, especially during times of stress to mitigate symptoms (Lehrer et al., 2002). Moreover, positive emotion may improve outcomes through its driver of healthy behaviors and treatment adherence, as well as physiologic functioning (Jenkins et al., 2021). A study of hope among pediatric patients showed that hope was a significant predictor for adherence to asthma treatment; the authors concluded that this construct needs further attention and research. Gratitude, one of the most commonly studied positive psychology constructs, has been recommended, along with hope optimism, and benefit finding, for children and adolescents with a spectrum of chronic conditions, including asthma, because of its early promising data (Kirschman et al., 2009). Overall, however, more rigorous research is needed to build a solid evidence base for PPIs in patients with asthma (Berg et al., 2007).

Conclusion

Traditional medical treatments often focus on symptom management, disease control, and prevention of complications. The clinical practice designed for positive health goes beyond this level of care to address the patient and their illness more holistically. By including positive psychology techniques integrated with lifestyle medicine treatments, positive health offers a promising approach for patients, promoting positive emotions, behaviors, and thoughts, and focusing on an individual's strengths and abilities to thrive despite illness. Associations have been shown between positive psychology constructs, such as meaning and social connection and improved wellbeing outcomes in chronically ill patients (Dezuttler et al. 2013). In turn, wellbeing may play a protective role during the course of physical illness. Lower stress has been associated with slower wound healing and greater survival (U.K. Department of Health Improvement Analytic Team, 2014).

Moreover, intentional interventions based on positive psychology, including gratitude journaling, mindfulness, positive reappraisal, solution-focused therapy, self-compassion practice, social support, and self-efficacy training, have been found to be effective in improving wellbeing and reducing symptoms of depression and anxiety, promoting self-esteem and self-efficacy among medically ill patients (Feig et al., 2019; Yan et al., 2020). Leading positive psychology researchers working in medical settings corroborate this potentially powerful role of PPIs in the context of illness (Moskowitz et al., 2019).

Specifically, positive self-talk, savoring positive experiences especially those associated with healthy behaviors, reframing negative thoughts, and focusing on strengths can help people with chronic diseases to adopt a greater sense of autonomy and self-efficacy, a positive attitude toward their illness, engage in healthy lifestyles, and improve their overall quality of life.

Although more research is needed, PPIs may also have a positive impact on physical health of the medically ill in several ways. They can reduce the deleterious effects of stress, improve immune system function (Cohen et al., 2003; Pressman & Black, 2012; Segerstrom & Miller, 2004; Segerstrom & Sephton, 2010), and lower disability due to pain (Müller et al., 2016). PPIs can improve biomarkers in some groups, such as those with coronary disease (Nikrahan et al., 2016) Hence, while there is still much to be learned about the relationship between positive psychology and physical health for patients with a wide spectrum of diseases, the literature suggests that positive psychology has the potential to, not only improve patients' mental and emotional wellbeing, but also physical health. When combined with lifestyle medicine, it can advance their positive health.

This powerful combination may treat diseases more effectively than each field can offer alone. The comprehensive approach of lifestyle medicine (e.g. healthy eating and physical activity) and positive psychology (e.g. gratitude, social connection, self-compassion) in the context of supportive environmental factors (such as the availability of walking paths and fresh fruit and vegetable markets) and communities with close social connections and supports can lead to positive health, not only for healthy populations but also for the medically ill. They can flourish despite their medical illnesses, at multiple levels, buffering mental health against the difficulties of managing chronic illness, bolstering mental and physical health, and building resources and capacity to thrive during future adversities (Waters et al., 2022).

As the field of positive health continues to evolve, it is likely that we will see more innovative interventions for individuals with chronic diseases, as well as studies of the short- and long-term outcomes of positive psychology approaches in lifestyle medicine and health care settings more broadly. Further research may more fully delineate the underlying mechanisms of action and the most effective interventions for specific chronic diseases and conditions and a wide spectrum of populations of varying demographics and cultures.

References

Alkozei, A., Smith, R., & Killgore, W. D. S. (2018). Gratitude and subjective well-being: A proposal of two causal frameworks. *Journal of Happiness Studies, 19*(5), 11519–1542. https://doi.org/10.1007/s10902-017-9870-1

Assarzadegan, M., & Raeisi, Z. (2019). The effectiveness of training based on positive psychology on quality of life and happiness of patients with type 2 diabetes. *Health Psychology, 8*(30), 97–116.

Bartlett, L., Buscot, M. J., Bindoff, A., & Chambers, R., & Hassed, C. (2021). Mindfulness is associated with lower stress and higher engagement in a large sample of MOOC participants. *Frontiers in Psychology, 12*, 724126. https://doi.org/10.3389/fpsyg.2021.724126

Bartlett, L., Martin, A., Neil, A. L., Mernish, K., Otahal, P., Kilpatrick, M., & Sanderson, K. (2019). A systematic review and meta-analysis of workplace mindfulness training randomized controlled trials. *Journal of Occupational Health Psychology, 24*(1), 108–126. https://doi.org/10.1037/ocp0000146.

Benkel, I., Arnby, M., & Molander, U. (2020). Living with a chronic disease: A quantitative study of the view of patients with a chronic disease on the change in life situation. *SAGE Open Medicine, 8*, 205031210910350. https://doi.org/10.1177/2050312120910350

Berg, C. J., Rapoff, M. A., Snyder, C. R., & Belmont, J. M. (2007). The relationship of children's hope to pediatric asthma treatment adherence. *Journal of Positive Psychology, 2*(3), 176–184. https://doi.org/10.1080/17439760701409629.

Black, D. S., & Slavich, G. M. (2016). Mindfulness meditation and the immune system: A systemic review of randomized controlled trials. *Annals of the New York Academy of Sciences, 1373*(1), 13–24. https://doi.org/10.1111/nyas.12998.

Boehm, J. K. (2021). Positive psychological well-being and cardiovascular disease: Exploring mechanistic and development pathways. *Soc Personal Psychol Compass, 15*(6), e12599. https://doi.org/10.1111/spc3.12599.

Boehm, J. K., & Kubzansky, L. D. (2012). The heart's content: The association between positive psychological well-being and cardiovascular health. *Psychological Bulletin, 138*(4), 655–691. https://doi.org/10.1037/a0027448.

Boehm, J. K., Trudel-Fitsgerald, C., Kivimaki, M., & Kubzansky, L. D. (2015). The prospective association between positive psychological wellbeing and diabetes. *Health Psychology, 34*(10), 1013–1021. https://doi.org/10.1037/hea0000200.

Boehm, J. K., Peterson, C., Kivimaki, M., Kubzansky, L. (2011). A prospective study of positive psychological wellbeing and coronary heart disease. *Health Psychology, 30*(3), 259–267. https://doi.org/10.1037/a0023124

Bohlmeijer, E., Prenger, R., Taal, E., & Cuijpers, P. (2010). The effects of mindfulness-based stress reduction therapy on mental health of adults with a chronic medical disease. *Journal of Psychosomatic Research, 68*(6), 539–44. https://doi.org/10.1016/j.jpsychores.2009.10.005.

Celano, C.M., Gianangelo, T. A., Millstein, R. A., Chung, W. J., Waxler, D. J., Park, E. R., & Huffman, J. C. (2018). A positive psychology-motivational interviewing intervention for patients with type 2 diabetes: Proof of concept trial. *International Journal of Psychiatry in Medicine, 54*(2), 97–114. https://doi.org/10.1177/0091217418791448.

Chakhssi, F., Kraiss, J. T., Sommers-Spijkerman, M., & Bohlmeijer, E. T. (2018). The effect of positive psychology interventions on well-being and distress in clinical samples with psychiatric or somatic disorders: A systematic review and meta-analysis. *BMC Psychiatry, 18*(1), 211. https://doi.org/10.1186/s12888-018-1739-2

Cohen, R., Bavishi, C., & Rozanski, A. (2016). Purpose in life and its relationship to all-cause mortality and cardiovascular events: A meta-analysis. *Psychosomatic Medicine, 8*(2), 122–133. https://doi.org/10.1097/PSY.0000000000000274.

Cohen, S., Doyle, W. J., Turner, R. B., Alper, C. M., & Skoner, D. P. (2003). Emotional style and susceptibility to the common cold. *Psychosomatic Medicine, 65*(4), 652–657. https://doi.org/10.1097/01.psy.0000077508.57784.da.

Cross, M. P., Hofschneider, L., Grimm, M., & Pressman, S. (2018). Subjective well-being and physical health. In E. Diener, S. Oishi, & L. Tay (Eds.), *Handbook of well-being* (pp. 472–489), DEF Publishers.

Dezutter, J., Casalin, S., Wachholtz, A., Lucyck, K., Hekking, J., & Vandewiele, W. (2013). Meaning in life: An important factors for the psychological well-being of chronically ill patients? *Rehabilitation Psychology, 58*(4), 334–341. https://doi.org/10.1037/a0034393

Diener, E., & Chan, M. Y. (2011). Happy people live longer: Subjective well-being contributes to health and longevity. *Applied Psychology: Health and Well-Being, 3*, 1–43. https://doi.org/10.1111/j.1758-0854.2010.01045.x

DiMatteo, M. R. (2004). Social support and patient adherence to medical treatment: A meta-analysis. *Health Psychology, 23*(2), 207–218. https://doi.org/10.1037/0278-6133.23.2.207.

Dubois, C. M., Lopez, O. V., Beale, E. E., Healy, B. C., Boehm, J. K., & Huffman, J. C. (2015). Relationships between positive psychological constructs and health outcomes in patients with cardiovascular disease: A systematic review. *International Journal of Cardiology, 195*, 265–280. https://doi.org/10.1016/j.ijcard.2015.05.121

Dubois, C. M., Millstein, R. M., Celano, C. M., Wexler, D. J., & Huffman, J. C. (2016). Feasibility and acceptability of a positive psychological intervention for patients with type 2 diabetes. *Primary Care Companion, 18*(3). https://doi.org/10.4088/PCC.15m01902

Emmons, R. A., & McCullough, M. E. (2003). Counting blessings versus burdens: An experimental investigation of gratitude and subjective well-being in daily life. *Journal of Personality and Social Psychology, 84*(2), 377–389. https://doi.org/10.1037/0022-3514.84.2.377.

Feig, E.H., Healy, B.C., Celano, C. M., Nikrahan, C. R., Moscowitz, J. T., & Huffman, J. (2019). Positive psychology interventions in patients with medical illness: What predicts improvement in psychological state? *International Journal of Well-Being, 9*(2), 27–40. https://doi.org/10.5502/ijw.v9i2.795

Gaffey, A. E., Rollman, B. L., & Burg, M. M. (2024). Strengthening the pillars of cardiovascular health: Psychological health is a crucial component. *Circulation, 149*, 641–643. https://doi.org/10.1161/CIRCULATIONAHA.123.066132

GBD 2019 Diseases and Injuries Collaborators. (2020). Global burden of 369 diseases and injuries in 204 countries and territories, 1990–2019: A systematic analysis for the global burden of disease study 2019. *The Lancet, 396*(10258), 1204–1222. https://doi.org/10.1016/S0140-6736(20)30925-9

Hajat, C., & Stein, E. (2018). The global burden of multiple chronic conditions: A narrative review. *Preventive Medicine Reports, 84*–293. https://doi.org/10.1016/j.pmedr.2018.10.008

Hendriks, T., Schotanus-Dijkstra, M., Hassankhan, A., de Jong, J., & Bohlmeijer, E. (2020). The efficacy of multi-component positive psychology interventions: A systematic review and meta-analysis of randomized controlled trials. *Journal of Happiness Studies. 21*, 357–290. https://doi.org/10.1007/s10902-019-00082-1

Hernandez, R., Cheung, E., Carnethon, M., Penedo, F. J., Moskowitz, J. T., Martinez, L., & Schuller, S. M. (2018). Feasibility of a culturally adapted positive psychological intervention for Hispanics/Latinos with elevated risk for cardiovascular disease. *Translational Behavioral Medicine, 8*(6), 887–897. https://doi.org/10.1093/tbm/iby045.

Howell, R. T., Kern, M. L., & Lyubomirsky, S. (2007). Health benefits: Meta-analytically determining the impact of wellbeing on objective health outcomes. *Health Psychology Review, 1*(1), 83136. https://doi.org/10.1080/17437190701492486

Huffman, J. C., Gilden, J., & Massey, C. N., Feig, W. H., Chung, W. J., Millstein, R. A., Brown, L., Giananeglo, Y., Healy, B. C., Wexler, D. J., Park, E. R., & Celano, C. M. (2021). A positive psychology-motivational interviewing intervention to promote positive affect and physical activity in type 2 diabetes; The BEHOLD-8 controlled clinical trial. *Psychosomatic Medicine, 82*(7), 641–649. https://doi.org/10.4081/hi.2011.e14

Huffman, J. C., Mastromauro, C. A., Boehm, J. K., Seabrook, R., Fricchione, G. L., & Denninger, J. W. (2011). Development of a positive psychology intervention for patients with acute cardiovascular disease. *Heart International, 6*(1), e14. https://doi.org/10.4081/hi.2011.e14.

Jasper, S. S., Datye, K., & Morrow, T., Sinsterra, M., LeStourgeon, L., Abadula, F., Bell, G. E., & Streisand, R. (2020) THRIVE! (2020). Positive psychology intervention to treat diabetes distress in teens with type 1 diabetes: Rationale and trial design. *Contemporary Clinicial Trials, 96,* 106086. https://doi.org/10.1016/j.cct.2020.106086

Jenkins, B. N., Moskowitz, J., Halterman, J. S., & Kain, Z. N. (2021). Appling theoretical models pf positive emotion to improve pediatric asthma: A positive psychology approach. *Pediatric Pulmonology, 56*(10), 3142–3147. https://doi.org/10.1002/ppul.25600.

Kabat-Zinn, J. (2003). Mindfulness-based stress reduction (MBSR). *Constructivism in the Human Sciences, 8*(2), 73. https://doi.org/10.1093/clipsy/bpg016.

Keng, S. L., Smoski, M. J., & Robins, C. J. (2011). Effects of mindfulness on psychological health: A review of empirical studies. *Clinical Psychology Review, 31*(6), 1041–1056. https://doi.org/10.1016/j.cpr.2011.04.006.

Kim, E. S., Chen, Y., & Nakamura, B. S., Ryff, C. D., & Vanderweele, T. J. (2022). Sense of purpose in life and subsequent physical, behavioral, and psychosocial health: An outcomes-wide approach. *American Journal of Health Promotion, 36*(1), 137–147. https://doi.org/10.1177/08901171211038545

Kim, E. S., Shiba, K., Boehm, J. K., & Kubzanzky, L. D. (2020). Sense of purpose in life and five health behaviors in older adults. *Preventive Medicine,*139, 106172. https://doi.org/10.1016/j.ypmed.2020.106172

Kim, E. S., Sun, J. K., Park, N., Kubzanzky, L. D., & Peterson, C. (2013a). Purpose in life and reduced risk of myocardial infarction among older US adults with coronary heart disease: A two-year follow-up. *Journal of Behavioral Medicine, 36*(2), 124–133. https://doi.org/10.1007/s10865-012-9406-4.

Kim, E. S., Sun, J. K., Park, N., & Peterson, C. (2013b). Purpose in life and reduced incidence of stroke in older adults: The health and retirement study. *Journal of Psychosomatic Research, 74*(5), 427–432. https://doi.org/10.1016/j.jpsychores.2013.01.013.

Kirschman, K .J. B., Johnson, R. J., & Roberts, M. C. (2009). Positive psychology for children and adolescents: Development, prevention, promotion. In Snyder, C. R. & Lopez, S. J. Handbook of Positive Psychology. Oxford University Press.

Kubzansky, L. D., Huffman, J. C., & Boehm, J. K., Hernandez, R., Kim, E. S., Koga, H. K., Feig, E. H., Lloyd-Jones, D. M., Seligman, M. E. P., & Labarthe, D. R. (2018). Positive psychological well-being and cardiovascular disease. JACC health promotion series. *Journal of the American College of Cardiology, 72*(12), 1382–1396. https://doi.org/10.1016/j.jacc.2018.07.042

Kubzansky, L. D., & Thurston, R. (2007). Emotional vitality and incident coronary heart disease. *Archives of General Psychiatry*, 64, 1393–1401. https://doi.org/10.1001/archpsyc.64.12.1393

Lehrer, P., Feldman, J., & Giardino, N., Song, H. S., & Schmaling, K. (2002). Psychological aspects of asthma. *Journal of Consulting and Clinical Psychology*, 70(3), 691–711. https://doi.org/10.1037/0022-006x.70.3.691

Levine, G. N., Cohen, B. E., Commodore-Mensah, Y., Fleury, J., Huffman, J. C., Khalid, U., Labarthe, D. R., Lavretsky, H., Michos, E. D., Spatz, E. S., & Kubzansky, L. D. (2021). Psychological health, well-being, and mind-heart-body connection: A scientific statement from the American Heart Association. *Circulation, 143*, e763–e783. https://doi.org/10.1161/CIR.0000000000000947

Liao, K. Y. H., & Weng, C. Y. (2018). Gratefulness and subjective wellbeing: Social connectedness and presence of meaning as mediators. *Journal of Counseling Psychology, 65*(3), 383–393. https://doi.org/10.1037/cou0000271.

Luszczynska, A., Benight, C. C., Cieslak, R., Kissinger, P., Reilly, K. H., & Clark, R. A. (2009). Self-efficacy mediates effects of exposure, loss of resources, and life stressors on posttraumatic distress among trauma survivors. *Applied Psychology Health and Well-Being. 1*(1), 73–90. https://doi.org/10.1111/j.1758-0854.2008.01005.x.

Maresova, P., Javanmardi, E., Barakovic, S., Husic, J. B., Tomsone, S., Krejcar, O., & Kuca, K., (2019). Consequences of chronic diseases and other limitations associated with old age – A scoping review. *BMC Public Health, 19*, 1431. https://doi.org/10.1186/s12889-019-7762-5

Massey, C. N., Feig, E. H., Duque-Serrano, L., & Huffman, J. C. (2017). Psychological wellbeing and type 2 diabetes. *Current Research in Diabetes & Obesity Journal, 4*(4), 555641. https://doi.org/10.19080/crdoj.2017.04.555641.

Masters, K. S., Shaffer, J. A., & Vagnini, K. M. (2020). The impact of psychological functioning in cardiovascular disease. *Current Atherosclerosis Reports, 22*, 51. https://doi.org/10.1007/s11883-020-00877-1

Mills, P. J., Redwine, L., & Wilson, K., Pung, M. A., Chinh, K., Greenberg, B. H., Lunde, O., Maisel, A., Raisingjani, A., Wood, A., & Chopra, D. (2015). The role of gratitude in spiritual wellbeing in asymptomatic heart failure patients. *Spirituality in Clinical Practice, 2*(1), 5–17. https://doi.org/10.1037/scp0000050

Moskowitz, J. T., Addington, E. L., & Cheung, E. O. (2019). Positive psychology and health: Well-being interventions in the context of illness. *General Hospital Psychiatry*, 61, 136–138. https://doi.org/10.1016/j.genhosppsych.2019.11.001

Moskowitz, J. T., Epel, E. S., & Acree, M. (2008). Positive affect uniquely predicts lower risk of mortality in people with diabetes. *Health Psychology, 27*(1S), S73–S82. https://doi.org/10.1037/0278-6133.27.1.S73.

Müller, R., Gerts, K. J., Molton, I. R., Terrill, A. L., Bombardier, C. H., Ehde, D. M., & Jensen, M. P. (2016). Effects of a tailored positive psychology intervention on wellbeing and pain in individuals with chronic pain and a physical disability. *The Clinical Journal of Pain, 32*(1), 32–44.

Nikrahan, G. R., Suarez, L., Asgari, K., Beach, S. R., Celano, C. M., Kalantari, M., Abedi, M. R., Etesampour, A., Abbas, R., & Huffman, J. C. C. M., & Kalantari, M., (2016). Positive psychology interventions for patients with heart disease: A preliminary randomized trial. *Psychosomatics, 57*(4), 348–358.

Park, N., Peterson, C., Szvarca, D., Vander Mole, R. J., & Collon, K. (2014). Positive psychology and physical health: Research and applications. *American Journal of Lifestyle Medicine, 10*(3), 200–206. https://doi.org/10.1177/1559827614550277.

Petersen, S., Göteborg, U., & Lundman, B. (2016). To be present in life and open to the future: A feasibility study of a mindfulness-based intervention for people with heart disease. *Scandinavian Journal of Caring Sciences, 30*(4), 740–748. https://doi. org/10.1111/scs.12311.

Pressman, S. D., & Black, L. L. (2012). Positive emotions and immunity. In S. C. Segerstrom (Ed.), *The Oxford handbook of psychoneuroimmunology* (pp. 92–104). Oxford University Press.

Redwine, L., Henry, B. L., Pung, M. A., Wilson, K., Chinh, K., Knight, B., Jain, S., Rutledge, T., Greenberg, B., Maisel, A., & Mills, P. J. (2016). A pilot randomized study of gratitude journaling intervention on HRV and inflammatory biomarkers in stage b heart failure patients. *Psychosomatic Medicine, 78*(6), 667–676. https://doi. org/10.1097/PSY.0000000000000316.

Sansone, R. A., & Sansone, L. A. (2010). Gratitude and wellbeing. *Psychiatry, 7*(11), 18–22.

Santiago, T., Geenan, R., & Jacobs, J. W., & Silva, J. A. P. (2015). Psychological factors associated with response to treatment in rheumatoid arthritis. *Current Pharmaceutical Design, 21*(2), 257–269. https://doi.org/10.2174/1381612820666140825 124755

Segerstrom, S. C., & Sephton, S. E. (2010). Optimistic expectancies and cell-mediated immunity: The role of positive affect. *Psychology Science, 21*(3), 448–455. https:// doi.org/10.1177/0956797610362061.

Segerstrom, S. S., & Miller, G. E. (2004). Psychological stress and the human immune system: A meta-analytic study of 30 years of inquiry. *Psychology Bulletin, 130*(4), 601–630. https://doi.org/10.1037/0033-2909.130.4.601.

Sin, N. L. (2017). The protective role of positive wellbeing in cardiovascular disease: Review of current evidence, mechanisms, and clinical implications. *Current Cardiology Reports, 18*(11), 106. https://doi.org/10.1007/s11886-016-0792-z.

Sirois, F. M. (2014). Positive psychological qualities and adjustment to arthritis. *OA Arthritis, 1*(2). ISSN 2052-9554.

Sirois, F. M., Kitner, R., & Hirsch, J. K. (2015). Self-compassion, affect, and health-promoting behaviors. *Health Psychology, 34*(6), 661–669. https://doi.org/10.1037/ hea0000158.

Sirois, F. M., & Wood, A. M. (2017). Gratitude uniquely predicts lower depression in chronic illness populations: A longitudinal study of inflammatory bowel disease and arthritis. *Health Psychology, 36*(2), 122–132. https://doi.org/10.1037/hea0000436.

Sneed, R. S., & Cohen, S. (2013). A prospective study of volunteerism and hypertension risk in older adults. *Health Psychology, 28,* 578–586. https://doi.org/10.1037/ a0032718

Stellar, J. E., John-Henderson, N., Anderson, C. L., Gordon, A. M., McNeil, G. D., & Keltner, D. (2015). Positive affect and markers of inflammation: Discrete positive emotions predict lower levels of inflammatory markers. *Emotion, 15*(2), 129–133. https://doi.org/10.1037/emo0000033.

Swain, N., Thompson, B. L., Gallgher, S., Paddison, J., & Mercer, S. (2020). Gratitude enhanced mindfulness (GEM): A pilot study of an internet-delivered program for self-management of pain and disability in people with arthritis. *Journal of Positive Psychology, 15*(3), 420–426. https://doi.org/10.1080/17439760.2019.1627397.

U.K. Department of Health Health Improvement Analytic Team. (2014). https://assets. publishing.service.gov.uk/media/5a75002ced915d502d6ccb51/Wellbeing_and_ Longevity.pdf

Van Cappellen, P., Rice, E. L., Catalino, L. I., & Fredrickson, B. L. (2017). Positive affective processes underlie positive health behavior change. *Psychol Health, 33*, 77–97. https://doi.org/10.1080/08870446.2017.1320798

Veenhoven, R. (1996). Happy life-expectancy: A comprehensive measure of quality-of-life in nations. *Social Indicators Research, 39*, 1–58. https://doi.org/10.1007/BF00300831

Waters, L., Algoe, S. B., Dutton, J., Emmons, R., Fredrickson, B.L., Heaphy, E., Moskowitz, J.T., Neff, K., Niemiec, R., Pury, C., Steger, M. (2022). Positive psychology in a pandemic: Buffering, bolstering, and building mental health. *Journal of Positive Psychology, 3*, 303–323. https://doi.org/10.1080/17439760.2021.1871945

Willroth, E.C., Mroczek, D. K., Hill, P. I. (2021). Maintaining sense of purpose in midlife predicts better physical health. *Journal of Psychosomatic Research, 145*, 110485 https://doi.org/10.1016/j.jpsychores.2021.110485

World Health Organization. *Noncommunicable diseases*. World Health Organization. September 16, 2022. https://www.who.int/news-room/fact-sheets/detail/noncommunicable-diseases

Xu, J., & Roberts, R. E. (2010). The power of positive emotions: It's a matter of life or death—Subjective well-being and longevity over 28 years in a general population. *Health Psychology, 29*, 9–19. https://doi.org/10.1037/a0016767

Xu, N. L., Zhao, S., Xue, H. X., Fu, A. Y., Zhang, T. Q., Huang, R., & Zhang, N. (2017). Associations of perceived social support and positive psychological resources with fatigue symptom in patients with rheumatoid arthritis. *PLoS One, 12*(3), e017393. https://doi.org/10.1371/journal.pone.0173293.

Yan, T., Chan, C.W.H., Chow, K.M., Zheng, W., & Sun, M. (2020). A systematic review of the effects of character strengths-based intervention on the psychological wellbeing of patients suffering from chronic illnesses. Journal of Advanced Nursing, 76(7), 1567–1580. https://doi.org/10.1111/jan.14356

Yi-Frazier, J. B., Hiliard, M., Cochrane, K., & Hood, K. K. (2012). The impact of positive psychology on diabetes outcomes: A review. *Psychology, 3*(12A), 1116–1124. https://doi.org/10.4236/psych.2012.312A165.

Yi-Frazier, J. P., Yaptangco, M., & Semana, S., Buscaino, E., Thompson, V., Cochrane, K., Tabile, M., Alving, E., & Rosenberg, A. R. (2015). The association of personal resilience with stress, coping, and diabetes outcomes in adolescents with type 1 diabetes: variable- and person-focused approaches. *Journal of Health Psychology, 20*(9), 1196–1206. https://doi.org/10.1177/1359105313509846

Zambrano, J., Celano, C. M., & Chung, W. J., Massey, C. N., Feig, E. H., Millstein, R. A. Healy, B. C., Wexler, D. J., Paek, E. R., Golden, J., & Huffman, J. C. (2020). Exploring the feasibility and impact of positive psychological-motivational interviewing interventions to promote positive affect and physical activity in type 2 diabetes: Design and methods from the BEHOLD-8 and BEHOLD-16 clinical trials. *Health Psychology and Behavioral Medicine, 8*(1), 398–422. https://doi.org/10.1080/21642850.2020.1815538

Zhang, A., Franklin, C., Currin-McCulloch, J., Park, S., & Kim, J. (2018). The effectiveness of strength-based, solution-focused brief therapy in medical settings: A systematic review and meta-analysis of randomized controlled trials. *Journal of Behavioral Medicine, 41*(1), 1–13. https://doi.org/10.1007/s10865-017-9888-1.

10 Clinical Applications for a Positive Health Practice

Chapter Overview

This chapter summarizes positive health clinical applications and describes how a healthcare practice can be redesigned to emphasize positive psychology with healthy lifestyles ("lifestyle medicine from the inside out") for achieving positive health. Positive health is a journey and a state of health and wellbeing that can be achieved by addressing traditional risk factors and boosting protective health factors based on the science of positive psychology in the context of other supportive factors in the biopsychosocial model, such as past traumas and adverse environmental conditions. Examples of tools are offered to inspire practitioners to take the early steps for adjusting their clinical approaches to promote and support positive health.

Introduction

A person-centered whole healthcare approach with emphasis on increasing positive health, not only treating illness, provides the foundation for the positive health clinical approach. The healthcare elements of assessment, treatment prescription, health coaching, monitoring progress, and follow-up can be redesigned through the lens of positive psychology in the context of positive health by emphasizing the desires and needs of the patient to achieve a comprehensive healthy lifestyle with positive activities.

Theoretical Underpinnings of a Positive Health Practice Model for Healthcare

Healthcare practices designed to help their patients achieve positive health may utilize the growing field of wellbeing theory and science and other positive psychology theoretical frameworks. Assessments include positive emotions as

DOI: 10.4324/9781003428909-10

they represent the core fuel for wellbeing change. The five-item World Health Organization (WHO-5) Wellbeing Index surveys for these drivers by asking about positive mood, vitality, and interest in life (Topp et al., 2015). Assessing positive experiences – social activities, accomplishments, and feel-good experiences, especially while doing healthy activities (Nezu & Nezu, 2018) harnesses the upward spiral theory of lifestyle change (Van Cappellen et al., 2018).

Positive health treatment includes practical positive psychology interventions (PPIs), activities that align with the PERMA model, to achieve emotional, mental, and physical wellbeing. The resulting improved psychological and subjective wellbeing (Hendriks et al., 2020) and increased positive emotions open the mind to solutions and advance problem-solving. The underpinnings of this process are described in the well-known broaden and build theory (Fredrickson, 2004, 2013).

Using the broaden-and-build-and related theories as a springboard, emotion-centered problem-solving therapy (ES-PST) has been developed. Based on empirical evidence, practical treatment applications of ES-PST for various clinic settings, patient populations, and clinical issues are available. Also, telehealth and community collaborative care models for integrating ES-PST (Nezu & Nezu, 2018) can be applied.

Positive healthcare approach can, additionally, utilize the widely implemented cognitive behavior therapy (CBT) process through reframing thoughts based on positive experiences. Positive CBT guides the patient to look for positive exceptions to problems, for example when they have less pain, and highlight those exceptions in their self-talk, as well as in their treatment solutions. In addition to the focus on positive emotions and experiences, another prominent feature of positive health practice is assisting patients to identify and use their strengths, character strengths (Niemiec & McGrath, 2019), personality-based strengths, and other personal strengths (Bannink & Peeters, 2021, Lianov, 2019) to act on and support recommended interventions and treatments.

Comparing Positive Healthcare with Traditional Healthcare and Lifestyle Medicine

As we review the clinical redesign to offer care that aims to achieve positive healthcare, a number of the distinctions between traditional and lifestyle medicine are described. Table 10.1 succinctly outlines these differences.

Positive Health Clinical Practice Starts with the Patient–Provider Interaction

In order to provide a successful approach to promoting positive health and disease treatment, practitioners first and foremost need to develop an effective therapeutic alliance, in which the person and what is most meaningful to them

Table 10.1 Differences between traditional medicine, lifestyle medicine, and positive health or "lifestyle medicine inside out" practice

	Traditional medicine	Lifestyle medicine	Positive health or "Lifestyle Medicine Inside Out"
Target Population	Patients with current illness	Patients with current illness or at risk for developing illness	General population
Assessment	Diagnostic tests	Lifestyle vital signs and diagnostic tests	Positive attributes, strengths, and level of life satisfaction and lifestyle vital signs
Treatment Goal	Symptom relief or stop disease progression	Disease remission or reversal	State of wellbeing achieved beyond reversal of traditional risk factors; ability to thrive and grow in the face of adversity
Treatment Interventions	Medications, procedures/ surgeries/ psychotherapy for symptom relief	Lifestyle interventions, health behavior changes	Lifestyle and PPIs, psychosocial interventions based on the biopsychosocial model
Prevention	Minimal to moderate focus on preventing disease and risk factors	Major focus on preventing disease and risk factors across the lifespan, primary focus on addressing and treating the root cause of disease	Major focus on preventing risk factors and promoting health protective factors based on positive psychology and the biopsychosocial model, along with healthy lifestyle change
Research	Advanced diagnostic tests and treatment procedures and addressing risk factors	Common underlying mechanisms/roots of disease and lifestyle interventions for a spectrum of diseases; effective methods of behavior change	Mechanisms of action of PPIs, the impact of specific PPIs in different populations, the role of positive emotions in physiologic improvements and behavior change, the impact of promoting a journey toward one's best self on disease prevention and treatment

Adaptation from Bannink & Peeters (2021)

takes center stage. The alliance builds on authentic connection based on the provider's understanding of the patient. This process requires connecting with the core values and complete biopsychosocial background of each patient. The comprehensive assessment and intervention approach collects and skillfully harnesses an understanding of personal values, work/career history, cultural, religious or spiritual beliefs, relationships, character and other personal strengths, and personality preferences (Brown & LaJambe, 2017).

Through the magic of an effective therapeutic alliance that connects the heart and soul of the patient and the provider, healing can begin. Positive interactions with patients based on positive psychology lead to an effective working relationship, support for health behavior change, improved emotional wellbeing, and direct physiologic benefits for both the patient and the provider (Major et al., 2018). This alliance opens the door to exploring the biopsychosocial constructs, as well as conducting mental health and positive psychology assessments, which can point to solutions and interventions that might otherwise remain hidden and serve as barriers to health behavior changes.

The therapeutic alliance allows for an "alternative dialogue" with the patient to shape the course of care toward positive health (Huber et al., 2022, p. 209). Many medical systems have built expectations by patients that they will receive medications and procedures as part of "good" care. Patients may be disappointed if they walk out without such concrete interventions. Lifestyle medicine is resigning healthcare to move away from these interventions and focus on health behavior change tactics and action plans as concrete steps. To focus on the latter, practitioners often hold alternative dialogues with patients about the efficacy of lifestyle changes and utilizing such changes as alternative treatments to medications and procedures. The person-centered whole health approach takes it further to focus on what the patient truly wants and their inner "why." Positive health practice goes even further to ensure that the alternative dialogue encompasses what is already going well, the patient's strengths, existing supports, and how to harness and build upon positive activities and social resources for ongoing thriving in the face of challenges well beyond the current medical condition.

Practical Clinical Applications and Supports for Positive Health

Implementing healthcare practice that emphasizes positive health includes adjusting each element of care through the lens of positive psychology and leveraging the entire healthcare team to support this approach. The clinical encounter is reframed to highlight what has been and is going well. The practitioner and other health team members serve as role models for noticing the positive during the visit. The clinical assessment includes measures of life satisfaction, hope, and other positive psychology constructs. The treatment prescriptions recommend positive activities, along with healthy lifestyle changes. When making treatment plans for patients with medical conditions that confer limitations, the practitioner focuses on what is feasible and how to leverage what the patient can still do to work toward personal goals. Treatment prescriptions include written instructions for positive psychology supports, such as the three S's – sharing, strengths, and savoring, as discussed later in the chapter. Alternatively, positive psychology supports are informally discussed with the patient when giving them the prescription. Coaching for health behavior change incorporates principles of positive psychology, including patient strengths, positive visioning, and integrating PERMA into health habit action plans. Follow-up on treatment can highlight and celebrate the patient's successes in order to align these changes as positive experiences and promote adherence (Lianov, 2019).

In a positive health-oriented practice, not only does the flow of care by the whole team emphasize positive constructs, but also the physical setting supports them. The healthcare workspace showcases positive images, images of kindness, and reminders about PPIs. Posters and waiting room videos spotlight the positive health values of the practice. For example, at the University of California San Francisco's Benioff Children's Hospital, a large digital monitor in the hallway to the cafeteria displays messages from the hospital leadership, including the wonders of practicing gratitude. One nonprofit organization is now dedicated to making available kindness images to health centers for digital displays. Although their results are not yet published, they are getting positive feedback regarding improved interactions between health workers and perceived positive experiences of patients.

Even a busy practitioner can adapt clinical flow processes to offer positive healthcare through team and digital support. Group visits/shared medical appointments, compared to one-on-one clinical encounters, allow more time to offer positive health educational programs and for patients to learn from positive experiences that are shared. Also, the practice may be more successful at helping patients achieve positive health when the entire health team is trained and learns how to infuse positive psychology strategies throughout the clinical flow. The nutritionist, medical fitness professional, and other team members in the clinic or in external programs can serve as "positive health paramedics" (Huber et al., 2022, p. 209). Outside referrals to like-minded local communities and online organizations, digital apps, and solutions that support positive health are additional ways to make this approach feasible and effective.

Moreover, self-care and informal care from volunteer peers and family can extend resources for better positive health-oriented care. Community programs can build a culture of activities that boost health and happiness to complement or supplement recommendations by the provider and help patients follow through with their action plans. Action for Happiness has been working with communities to transform them into positive health environments through the dissemination of key principles to happier living (giving, relating, exercising, mindful awareness, trying out new things, setting goals, finding ways to bounce back, looking for what's good, acceptance of who you are, and being a part of something meaningful), education, a calendar of events, and practical tools that can be easily implemented (https://actionforhappiness.org). The Act-Belong-Commit (ABC) Coalition in Australia that encourages individuals to be proactive about their mental health is another community program that highlights positive psychology constructs, such as helping others by volunteering and mentoring and engaging in activities that promote socialization to contribute to a culture of wellbeing outside of healthcare settings (Egger et al., 2011).

The issue of time management is an important one to consider for all clinical practices, and positive health-oriented practices are no exception. In fact, lack of time is a common barrier to these positive health approaches cited by practitioners. Many readers may be familiar with the four quadrants of time management: important and urgent non important and urgent, important and not urgent, and not important and not urgent. Of course, most of us can easily let go of the latter quadrant. However, we are challenged to let go of urgent tasks, whether they are important or not important. Practicing positive health in care calls for letting go of urgent, but not important matters of care (such as inappropriate referrals, reactive requests for help, and additional work due to insufficient triage). Instead, we need to focus on the important, but not urgent quadrant, such as holding alternative dialogues, helping patients develop proactive action plans for flourishing, and developing patient strengths lists (Huber et al., 2022, p. 146).

A health system can choose to undertake positive health transformation and help advance the positive health movement through the leadership and assistance of organizations like the Global Positive Health Institute (GPHI). The GPHI is working to inspire and train leaders and champions across a number of countries. The International Positive Psychology Association's Positive Health and Wellbeing Division through its educational offerings to health professionals and the American College of Lifestyle Medicine through its new work to examine the role of meaning, purpose, and spirituality in health – are delving further into ways to transform healthcare toward positive health. If a practitioner who is passionate about this type of healthcare practice finds limited interest in such change in their organization, they can adapt smaller, more manageable changes in how they approach patients. That small change might simply entail a shift in attention to what is going well for the patient and using the patient's strengths to springboard successful treatment action plans. Table 10.2 provides suggestions of positive health tools and strategies for each element of healthcare.

Lifestyle Medicine Competencies: Key Clinical Processes with Positive Health Expansion

Many of the lifestyle medicine competencies in the section on key clinical processes can be expanded to encompass positive healthcare. Table 10.3 outlines these useful expansions.

Table 10.2 Integrating positive health into the flow of healthcare

Healthcare element	Positive health practice tools and strategies – Examples
Intake	Identification of character strengths (viacharacter.org), key values, positive goals, social supports, joyful activities, current and past wellbeing practices, and accomplishments (e.g. meditation or gratitude practice)
Assessment	Satisfaction with Life Scale, Flourishing Scale, Hope Scale
Intervention Prescription	PPI prescription templates (examples listed in Chapters 3 to 8)
Intervention Action Planning	Three S's – sharing, strengths, savoring (examples in Chapters 3 to 8)
Health Coaching	Appreciative Inquiry, PERMA integrated questions (examples in Chapters 3 to 8)
Follow-up and Monitoring	Emphasize action plan successes (partial or complete), healthy rewards
Clinical Setting – Structure	Website, posters, and digital media in clinics displaying kindness images and positive psychology messages and constructs
Clinical Setting – Process, Mindset, and Culture	Gratitude shared during health team huddles, positive orientation of patient and coworker questions (e.g. what has gone well?)
Referrals	External health coaches and psychologists who emphasize positive psychology; community classes (e.g. Action for Happiness and digital apps, e.g. My Happy Avatar)

Table 10.3 Integrating positive health into lifestyle medicine: Competencies for key clinical processes in lifestyle medicine

Lifestyle medicine competency	Positive health expansion
Integrate lifestyle vital signs into components of the patient history and physical exam	Conduct brief assessments of life satisfaction and positive activity habits
Analyze and implement evidence-based clinical practice guidelines relevant to lifestyle medicine for the prevention, treatment, and reversal of chronic diseases	Utilize positive health approaches to assist patients in follow-through with treatment recommendations of practice guidelines
Describe the treatment of disease with the lifestyle medicine pillars as compared with medication	Integrate positive psychology approaches (mindsets and activities) into treatment with the lifestyle medicine pillars for successful behavior change and for physiologic benefits (protective health factors)

(Continued)

Table 10.3 (Continued)

Lifestyle medicine competency	Positive health expansion
Demonstrate how to screen, diagnose, treat, and monitor a lifestyle-related disease and provide lifestyle medicine – focused anticipatory guidance	Apply positive health strategies, such as highlighting positive emotions and experiences, in anticipatory guidance
Discuss strategies for a clinical practice to access and implement the use of local, national, and global resources	Harness credible resources in positive psychology, such as those offered by the University of Pennsylvania, the Benson Henry Institute, and the International Positive Psychology Association
Describe the key strategies for leveraging inter-professional teams to enhance health behavior change interventions	Engage in positive patient and coworker interactions and jointly emphasize positive psychology principles (e.g. emphasis on patient strengths, in effective interprofessional care teams)
Examine how group visits and telehealth can optimize lifestyle medicine treatment encounters	Incorporate positive health education, and positive interactions and activities into group visits; harness social connection benefits provided by members of the group
Create and utilize data from office systems, such as electronic health records with lifestyle medicine guidance, in clinical decisions and care, including tracking screening frequency, test results, referrals, and recommended follow-up	Design systems that monitor and utilize data on each patient's "whys" patient strengths and positive biopsychosocial supports
Analyze the evidence for collaborative and chronic care models on improved lifestyle outcomes	Analyze and apply positive healthcare models, such as the spider web model by the Institute of Positive Health (which includes bodily functions, mental wellbeing, meaningfulness, quality of life, participation, and daily functioning)
Discuss successful primary care and office-based models for lifestyle modification	Discuss positive health models that (e.g. the Institute of Positive Health spider web model) provide a broader view of health with interventions that support the ability to adapt in the face of challenges and build on personal personal meaningful goals and strengths
Design a quality improvement project for lifestyle medicine clinical practice, using tools, such as Plan-Do-Study-Act (PDSA) cycles	Implement PDSA cycles to apply and test positive health strategies in clinical practice

(Continued)

Table 10.3 (Continued)

Lifestyle medicine competency	Positive health expansion
Explain the principles of evidence-based medicine and their application to lifestyle medicine	Apply evidence-based medicine principles to the study and application of positive health and positive psychology integration into lifestyle medicine
Describe methods of assessing the effectiveness of interventions, such as patient activation measures and the therapeutic alliance measures	Describe interventions that assess the effectiveness of positive psychology strategies to increase patient activation and boost the therapeutic alliance

Key Role of Positive Psychology in Health Coaching

Health behavior change is the foundation for improved outcomes in lifestyle medicine and positive health. Much literature is available on coaching theory, science, and practice covering a variety of techniques. However, the heart of effectively helping patients make changes relies on collaboration and positive psychology approaches. Therefore, all positive health models of care lean heavily on this component of care.

The field of health coaching has been a front-runner in healthcare for implementing positive psychology. As health coaches guide individuals to adopt health behaviors that address underlying causes of disease, they weave in positive future visioning, appreciative inquiry, and elements of PERMA (Lianov, 2019), as well as effective use of strengths (McQuaid et al., 2019).

During motivational interviewing, the pros and cons of making change are explored and, in a positive health approach, the patient is nudged to emphasize how the desired change will help them achieve positive goals rather than avoid negative consequences. Moreover, the desired lifestyle can be connected to hope – a positive forward driver for perseverance and change (Hibbard et al., 2010).

When coaching a health behavior change, one can connect the desired behavior with as many of the elements of PERMA as possible (Falecki et al., 2019, Lianov, 2019) to promote positive emotions, leveraging nonconscious motivation for the behavior, as described in the upward spiral or lifestyle change (Van Cappellen et al., 2018).

P—Positive emotions: Savor positive feelings that arise when doing the behavior

E—Engagement (Flow): Do the activity in ways that make you lose track of time and surroundings and become mindful of the present positive experience

R—Relationships: Identify how the activity can be done with others and increase social interactions

M—Meaning: Pay attention to how the behavior aligns with your values and life purpose and what feels meaningful

A—Achievement: Reflect on how progress toward the behavioral goal gives you a sense of accomplishment.

Empirical studies show that these kinds of approaches during health behavior coaching are associated with greater behavioral changes, including among medically ill patients. For example, PPIs have been successfully used to promote health behavior change in acute coronary syndrome (Celano et al., 2018). Hence, leading authors in health coaching emphasize the role of positive psychology and a collaborative approach – which can boost a therapeutic alliance and positivity resonance – for successful results (Biswas-Diener, 2012; Kaufman, 2006; Olsen & Nesbitt, 2010; Reynolds et al., 2019). Table 10.4 showcases how the health behavior change section of the lifestyle medicine competencies can be expanded with positive health principles.

Table 10.4 Integrating positive health into lifestyle medicine: Fundamentals of health behavior change

Lifestyle medicine competency	*Positive health expansion*
Summarize health behavior change theories, such as the health belief model, the social learning theory, and the transtheoretical model (TTM), and their application to lifestyle medicine practice	Summarize positive psychology principles in health behavior change, with emphasis on positive emotions as a key driver for behavior change
Demonstrate key elements of conducting a patient assessment within the TTM and collaborate to develop stage-matched responses	Incorporate positive psychology constructs into the stage-matched responses that validate the patients' strengths and progress toward goals
Apply the process of building effective and therapeutic alliances with patients that foster their personal growth	Build therapeutic alliances through positive interactions with patients, such as highlighting positive moments during the clinical encounter, pointing out patient strengths, and praising progress toward goals
Explain how to collaborate with your patients to promote health behavior changes	Collaborate with patients to promote health behavior change with positive psychology mindsets and activities, such as positive future visioning, aligning activities with meaningful values, and using character strengths

(Continued)

Table 10.4 (Continued)

Lifestyle medicine competency	Positive health expansion
Apply motivational interviewing, cognitive behavioral, health coaching, and positive psychology techniques	Utilize positive psychology techniques when coaching healthy behaviors; foster positive emotions with PERMA elements during targeted behaviors
Summarize the evidence to support the use of behavior change techniques in clinical practice	Summarize the evidence for positive psychology applications in health behavior coaching
Use the skills of open inquiry, reflection, and empathy to develop and maintain a therapeutic alliance	Apply positive psychology skills in building the therapeutic alliance, such as promoting positivity resonance and conducting appreciative inquiry
Describe the impact of positive emotions on the success of health behavior change	Describe the role of positive emotions during a desired behavior in the upward spiral theory of lifestyle change; describe the reciprocal, reinforcing link of positive emotions and the major lifestyle medicine pillars
Develop patient-centered, written action plans based on the appropriate stage of change of the TTM	Develop action plans with positive activities – based on patient culture, interests, and personality; ensure action plans highlight the shifting attention to positive emotions during the desired behavior
Summarize the process of follow-up for ongoing lifestyle change progress, including building patient self-efficacy and relapse prevention	Praise progress toward desired goals, encourage self-praise, and healthy self-rewards for progress; reframe self-talk about a lapse or relapse into authentic support and with self-compassion
Describe the factors that support sustained behavior change	Describe the role of positive emotions in sustaining behavior change, describe vantage resources in the upward spiral of lifestyle change that support successful and sustainable change
Explain the role of family and other support to initiate and maintain health behavior change	Explain how social connections and relationships during desired behaviors can boost positive emotions to reinforce those behaviors
Manage disruptions to the therapeutic alliance	Explain how positive interactions boost positive emotions and positivity resonance and can contribute to building and rebuilding the therapeutic alliance
Identify patient resources for sustainable behavior change in relation to the pillars of lifestyle medicine	Identify patient resources on how to leverage positive activities – leading to positive emotions – in making behavior changes for each pillar of a healthy lifestyle change

Case Study of Reframing the Clinical Approach Toward Positive Health

Hannah, a 65-year-old patient with pre-diabetes and mild depression who lives alone is seen in the clinic every three months. Her hemoglobin A1c has been consistent at 6.1 and her blood pressure has been increasing, today at 142/88. She is making little progress with a health coach to adopt a plant-predominant whole-food eating pattern and to increase her total weekly walking time.

What are examples of initial steps in a traditional medical practice versus a lifestyle medicine practice and a positive healthcare practice?

Traditional medical approach: Offer her medications, an antihypertensive and a selective serotonin reuptake inhibitor, and arrange for her to continue working with a health coach. In many cases, she may have already been prescribed medications in addition to the lifestyle change recommendation.

Lifestyle medicine approach: Assess her biopsychosocial background (including past and ongoing trauma and current social-emotional environment) and develop a patient-centered action plan to increase her social connections and explore other ways to help support her in making health behavior changes; help her restructure her healthy eating and physical activity plan to one that she has self-confidence she can achieve; inquire about her interest in an intensive lifestyle intervention program.

Positive health approach: Explore what matters to the patient and what is meaningful to her; focus on what is already going well and the positive activities in which she currently engages; develop an action plan for positive activities that she expresses as her "personal why" goals, including social, volunteer and spiritual/religious activities. Identify her character and other personal strengths and develop a plan to leverage them to succeed in these activities. Inquire about her interest and readiness level to adjust her healthy eating and physical activity plan. You might to do so after she conducts positive activities to promote emotional wellbeing and capacity to follow-through.

Perspectives in Practicing Lifestyle Medicine from the Inside Out – The Clinical Encounter

As has been emphasized in this chapter, even without a significant increase in clinical practice time, most health professionals can proactively adopt the fundamental elements of positive health, such as starting a clinical encounter by asking "What matters to you in improving your health, wellbeing and life?" Professionals in lifestyle medicine, general medical care, and in specialty care, such as cardiology, can practice through the lens of empowering the patients and encouraging them to use their personal strengths, engage in positive activities as part of their healthy lifestyle plan, and savor positive experiences during a desired health behavior. For patients who have experienced adversity, helping them to reframe their situation and look for what is feasible and meaningful in the light of past and current trauma is essential. To support this work, medical practitioners can also refer to other health professionals, such as behavioral health workers, health coaches and nurses, either on their team or externally. These health professionals can conduct alternative dialogues with the patients, help identify their strengths, and develop action plans that leverage strengths and set goals to add or increase positive activities as part of the comprehensive lifestyle treatment plan. They can refer to community resources, online programs, and apps to conduct this approach with effectiveness and efficiency.

Despite this framework for embracing positive health, some physicians and health professionals may not be inspired to practice this way, preferring to focus their clinical time on their medical specialty area. As healthcare evolves, it is possible that the implementation of both lifestyle medicine and positive health may be integrated by a segment of providers rather than widely. The lifestyle medicine intensivists will tackle the deep dive of working with patients on intensive healthy lifestyle changes, while other health professionals will apply a few elements of this care.

The same trajectory may occur with positive-health oriented healthcare. The Dutch propose the T-shaped professional model, which trains two groups of health professionals. The first group consists of professionals who have disease-specific expertise and hence implement the basics of the positive health model. The second group fully implements the whole-person approach toward positive health. The latter identifies patient strengths and assesses life satisfaction, positive emotions, mental health, and social and emotional wellbeing as well as the physical condition, provides coaching with an emphasis on and full integration of positive psychology principles, and collaborates with the patient to develop positive health action plans (Huber et al., 2022, p. 39).

Practitioners need to do some self-reflection about what kind of clinical practice best suits their goals, interests, and personalities. Some may choose to leave this type of care to colleagues. Others may choose to dive into a total positive health practice transformation, especially when it aligns with their overarching professional aims. The energy from engaging in, leading and championing a healthcare practice well-aligned with positive health values opens up the problem-solving capacity to address and overcome system and other barriers that may arise. Most health professionals will likely choose to implement a few of the suggestions in this text that can be easily implemented and allow them to engage in clinical practice with a joyful heart.

Conclusion

Healthcare practice can be redesigned to focus on a person-centered whole-health approach with an emphasis on integrating positive psychology into all major elements of care. Prioritizing the positive health continuum when necessary and appropriate can frame the approach to treating disease in ways that are relevant and meaningful to the patient. That approach will help them on the journey toward a state of positive health, a state of wellbeing achieved when addressing positive psychology factors that serve as health protective factors, along with a comprehensive healthy lifestyle in the context of supportive factors in the biopsychosocial model. Positive health is a springboard for the capacity to flourish by adjusting self-care and healthcare in response to changing and challenging environments on the road of life so that individuals can function as their best-selves.

References

Bannink, F., & Peeters, F. (2021) *Practicing positive psychiatry*. Hogrefe Publishing Corporation, pp. 17, 23–25, 29, 33.

Biswas-Diener, R. (2012). *Practicing positive psychology coaching: Assessment, activities and strategies for success*. John Wiley & Sons.

Brown, F., & LaJambe, C. (2017). *Positive psychology and wellbeing, applications for enhanced living*. Cognella Academic Publishing.

Celano, C. M., Albanese, A. M., Millstein, R. A., Mastromauro, C. A., Chung, W.-J., Campbell, K. A., Leglet, S. R., Park, E. R., Healy, B. C., Collins, L. M., Januzzi, J. L., & Huffman, J. C. (2018). Optimizing a positive psychology intervention to promote health behaviors following an acute coronary syndrome: The positive emotions after acute coronary events III (PEACE-III) randomized factorial trial. *Psychosomatic Medicine, 80*(6), 526–534. https://doi.org/10.1097/PSY.0000000000000584.

Egger, G., Binns, A., & Rossner, S. (2011). *Lifestyle medicine, managing diseases of lifestyle in the 21ˢᵗ century* (2nd ed.). The McGraw-Hill Companies.

Falecki, D., Leach, C., & Green, S. (2019). PERMA-powered coaching: Building foundations for a flourishing life. In S. Green & S. Palmer (Eds.), *Positive psychology coaching in practice* (pp. 103–120). Routledge.

Fredrickson, B. L. (2004). The broaden-and-build theory of positive emotions. *Philosophical Transactions of the Royal Society of London, 359*, 1367–1377. https://doi.org/10.1098/rstb.2004.1512

Fredrickson, B. L. (2013). Positive emotions broaden and build. *Advances in Experimental Social Psychology., 47*, 1–53. https://doi.org/10.1037/0003-066x.56.3.218

Hendriks, T., Schotanus-Dijkstra, M., & Aabiden, H. (2020). The efficacy of multicomponent positive psychology interventions: A systematic review and meta-analysis of randomized controlled trails. *Journal of Happiness Studies, 21*(1), 357–390. https://doi.org/10.1007/s10902-019-00082-1.

Hibbard, J., Lawso, K., Moore, M., & Wolever, R. (2010). *Three pillars of health coaching, patient activation, motivational interviewing and positive psychology*. Healthcare Intelligence Network.

Huber, M., Jung, H. P., van den Brekel-Dijkstra, K. (2022). *Handbook: Positive Health in Primary Care, The Dutch Example.* The Netherlands, Bohn Stafleu van Loghum.

Kaufman, C. (2006). Positive psychology: The science at the heart of coaching. In D. Stober & A. Grant (Eds.), *Evidence-based coaching: Putting best practices to work for your clients* (pp. 219–253). John Wiley & Sons.

Lianov, L. (2019). *Roots of positive change, optimizing health care with positive psychology.* American College of Lifestyle Medicine and HealthType LLC.

Major, B. C., Le Nguyen, K. D., Lundberg, K. B., & Fredrickson, B. L. (2018). Well-being correlates of perceived positivity resonance: Evidence from trait and episode-level assessments. *Personality and Social Psychology Bulletin, 44*(12), 1631–1647. https://doi.org/10.1177/0146167218771324.

McQuaid, M., Niemiec, R., & Doman, F. (2019). A character strengths-based approach to positive psychology. Positive psychology coaching for health and wellbeing. In S. Green & S. Palmer (Eds.), *Positive psychology coaching in practice* (pp. 57–65). Routledge.

Nezu, A. M., & Nezu, C. M. (2018). *Emotion-centered problem-solving therapy, treatment guidelines.* Springer Publishing Company.

Niemiec, R. M., & McGrath, R. E. (2019). *The power of character strengths, an official guide from the VIA institute on character.* VIA Institute on Character.

Olsen, J. M., & Nesbitt, B. J. (2010). Health coaching to improve healthy lifestyle behaviors: An integrative review. *American Journal of Health Promotion, 25*(1), e1–e12. https://doi.org/10.4278/ajhp.090313-LIT-101.

Reynolds, R., Palmer, S., & Green, S. (2019). Positive psychology coaching for health and wellbeing. In S. Green, & S. Palmer (Eds.), *Positive psychology coaching in practice* (pp. 95–109). Routledge.

Topp, C. W., Østergaard, S. D., Søndergaard, S., & Bech, P. (2015). The WHO-5 well-being index: A systematic review of the literature. *Psychotherapy and Psychosomatics, 84*(3), 167–176. https://doi.org/10.1159/000376585.

Van Cappellen, P., Rice, E. L., Catalino, L. I., & Fredrickson, B. L. (2018). Positive affective processes underlie positive health behavior change. *Psychology & Health, 33*(1), 77–97. https://doi.org/10.1080/08870446.2017.1320798.

Epilogue
A Call to Action

From the perspective of busy and overwhelmed healthcare professionals, the idea of making changes in clinical care to accommodate positive psychology approaches may at first glance seem inappropriate. That view may be the case, especially among those who are unfamiliar with this science which focuses on much more than increasing happiness or always being positive. Through the science and suggested practices shared in this text, our hope is that readers grasp, not only the relevance and feasibility of integrating positive psychology into care (by leveraging the health team and digital resources), but also the foundational role this kind of approach plays in achieving goals central to health and wellbeing. Positive psychology is an approach to thriving that embraces our humanity and a full range of emotions with science-based, compassionate strategies. When combined with healthy lifestyle habits, we build positive health.

While much research remains ahead, we have an urgency to act using the science and tools available today. By harnessing healthy lifestyles and positive psychology approaches, we can make progress along the continuum of positive health. The medical field of lifestyle medicine is especially well poised to do this because it is centered on six healthy lifestyle pillars that can be effectively facilitated by and intertwined with positive psychology – leading to benefits for all major elements of well-being in prevention and treatment. Moreover, the positive health approach builds resilience and can even promote growth in the face of adversity. Now more than ever, as humans collectively face the multi-level, interwoven complex crises of increasing societal polarization, violence, wars, isolation, uncertainties of the impact of rapid technology changes such as artificial intelligence, and the existential threat to the planet, we need to take care of ourselves from a center of heart and wisdom. Health providers with the assistance and support of the entire healthcare team need to do the same for their patients.

Of course, achieving full flourishing relies on much more than what can be done by the individual and the healthcare team; it requires communal action so that we can flourish personally, socially, and in a healthy environment. That being said, in the current milieu, the role of the health care professions is evolving, as seen in programs such as the Veteran's Affairs Whole Health program offering person-centered care. We can no longer, in good conscience, continue to focus on individuals and the reductionistic approach of diagnostic tests and treatments offered in isolation of the whole individual and his environment, expecting good outcomes for patients and satisfaction as health professionals. Although many healthcare systems and reimbursement mechanisms have yet to catch-up to this evolving role, the call to action is upon us. We must redesign our approach to be able to thrive in our rapidly evolving world.

We can start by taking care of ourselves with self-compassion and engaging in interaction with patients, coworkers, friends, family, and the community with love, focusing on what matters most to them. Many definitions of love are embraced; the one that seems appropriate here is "the pursuit of the wellbeing of the other." That's the ultimate role of each health professional and all of us in daily life, as our well-being has to embrace our interdependence. Let's move forward with this in mind to advance flourishing together for humanity.

Index

Note: Locators in *italics* represent figures and **bold** indicate tables in the text.